Everything's Okay

100% OF THIS BOOK'S PROFITS WILL BE DONATED TO
THE CHILDREN'S HOSPITAL OF PHILADELPHIA

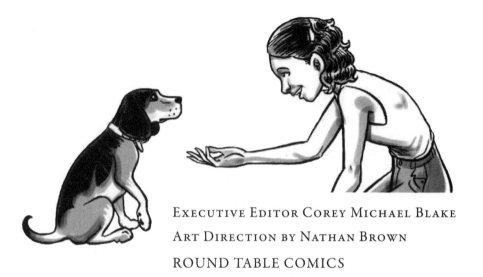

Executive Editor Corey Michael Blake

Art Direction by Nathan Brown

ROUND TABLE COMICS

Everything's Okay

BASED ON THE ORIGINAL MEMOIR BY

ALESIA SHUTE

ILLUSTRATED BY
NATHAN LUETH

GRAPHIC ADAPTATION BY
NADJA BAER

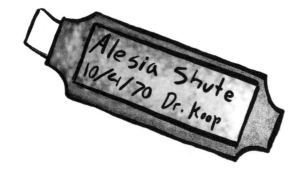

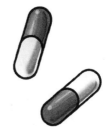

© 2011 Writers of the Round Table Press and Alesia Shute
Round Table Comics

@RNDTABLECOMICS
WWW.ROUNDTABLECOMICS.COM

Round Table Companies
1670 Valencia Way
Mundelein, IL 60060
USA

Phone: 815-346-2398

First Edition: Sept 2011
ISBN: 978-1-61066-014-3

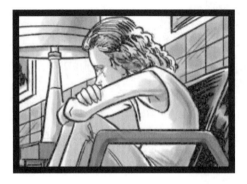

Printed in Canada

I HAVE MET WITH HER OTHER DOCTORS AND WE ALL AGREE: ALESIA NEEDS A SURGERY THAT WE NORMALLY DO NOT PERFORM ON CHILDREN, BUT WE HAVE NO CHOICE. OTHERWISE, SHE WILL ONLY GET WORSE AND WILL PROBABLY NOT LIVE PAST THE AGE OF 16.

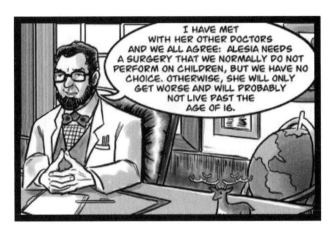

"Life affords no greater responsibility, no greater privilege, than the raising of the next generation."
- C. Everett Koop

Foreword

I will never forget January 24, 2007... the day my life changed forever – the day I was told my unborn baby had a stroke in utero.

Like many couples, my husband and I had difficulty conceiving a child and we'd had a stillborn baby years earlier, so my doctors were monitoring me closely this time around. I was 28 weeks pregnant and had no major problems. In fact, before then – before that moment when they broke the news to me – I never even knew an unborn baby could have a stroke.

After hearing them tell me that day that my baby would have right-sided weakness, developmental delays and cerebral palsy, I went home from Children's Hospital of Philadelphia (CHOP), curled up in my bed, and cried uncontrollably. The news completely devastated my husband and me. The fear of the unknown and of what lay ahead was so scary.

My son RJ was born two months later on March 22 and began life in the hospital neonatal intensive care unit (NICU) with tubes, IVs, doctors, tests, and medicines. He had three cardiac arrests before he was five months old. The last time he "coded" in the NICU – on Father's Day that year – the doctor told me RJ would never walk, talk, eat or see. I worried every day whether he would live to see the next. All my hopes and dreams for him seemed lost, and my heart ached not knowing what the future would bring. As a mother, watching him suffer and knowing I could not make him better was one of the hardest things I've had to do. I felt helpless, alone and afraid. My husband and I never could have prepared for the challenges that we would face on a daily basis, which caused tremendous physical, mental, emotional and financial strain on our marriage.

I met Alesia on a Sunday in October at a craft fair festival. She had set up a table for her foundation and was selling raffle tickets and copies of her book, with all proceeds going to CHOP. As we talked, she told my husband and me that she was speaking to a stroke support group for parents the following Tuesday. Funny how I was supposed to attend that support group meeting but had already decided not to go. After I met Alesia, however, I knew I had to hear her story. Things work in mysterious ways – I believe we were meant to meet that day at the festival.

I went to the meeting on Tuesday to see Alesia but never dreamed she would change my life the way she did. At the time, I was struggling with a special needs baby that missed every developmental milestone. RJ did not roll over until he was almost one year old, did not crawl until he was two and a half, and did not walk until he was three and a half. With ten therapies a week, I was exhausted and depressed. I felt alone and like a failure at times because of the daily challenges. Yet listening to her talk about her own childhood cancer touched my heart. It gave me a reason to believe good things were possible.

During that meeting, I received a copy of Alesia's book titled "Everything's Okay". After reading it that night, I was full of mixed emotions and cried aloud. Just like RJ, her childhood was anything but normal – it was full of pain and hospitals, and she had endured several operations. But she never gave up hope and never lost her determination. She did not let her sickness knock her down. Alesia was a fighter who was determined to beat her cancer. As RJ grows up and encounters increasingly difficult days, I know Alesia's story will forever leave a positive mark on his life.

Alesia has touched many families who are looking for hope during their struggle with a sick child, and I believe her story will give you the same strength and inspiration that it has given them and that it gave me. Knowing that she survived cancer and seeing the great things she is doing today made me realize there is a light at the end of my tunnel and that everything can and will be okay. She let me know that I am not alone and that I have to keep moving forward – even when I have a bad day. I now have the courage to face tomorrow and the day after that and the day after that. And it's alright if I fall down... I will eventually get back up!

"Everything's Okay" will show you that there is, indeed, a light at the end of your tunnel, too. You may not be able to see it; you just have to believe you will get there someday!

Lisa Mousley
Mother of a Pediatric Stroke Survivor

GET WELL
ICE

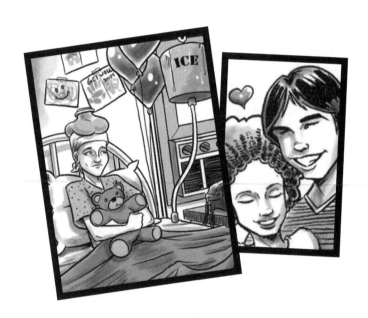

We all know people whose suffering has affected not only their own life, but also the lives of those around them. Such was the case when a serious childhood illness forever changed me, my siblings, parents, and friends, and had a profound effect on the adult relationships I later developed.

"Everything's Okay," the original full-length book about my experiences, has gone well beyond telling the story my life; it has helped countless people who are bravely caring for a sick family member.

Round Table Comics has now transformed "Everything's Okay" into a comic book version that visually depicts the challenges I faced and the triumphs I have celebrated throughout my life as I reached new milestones. I hope you draw strength and courage from these events and that this edition inspires you to wake up each day and say, "I can do this!"

My family and friends, especially my son and husband, have been the "Wind beneath my Wings" as I worked with Round Table Comics on this exciting new project. All profits from the sale of this version of "Everything's Okay" will go to The Children's Hospital of Philadelphia, so THANK YOU on behalf of them.

Enjoy!
Alesia Shute

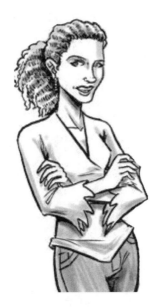

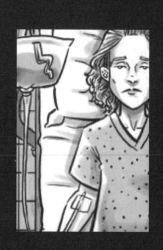

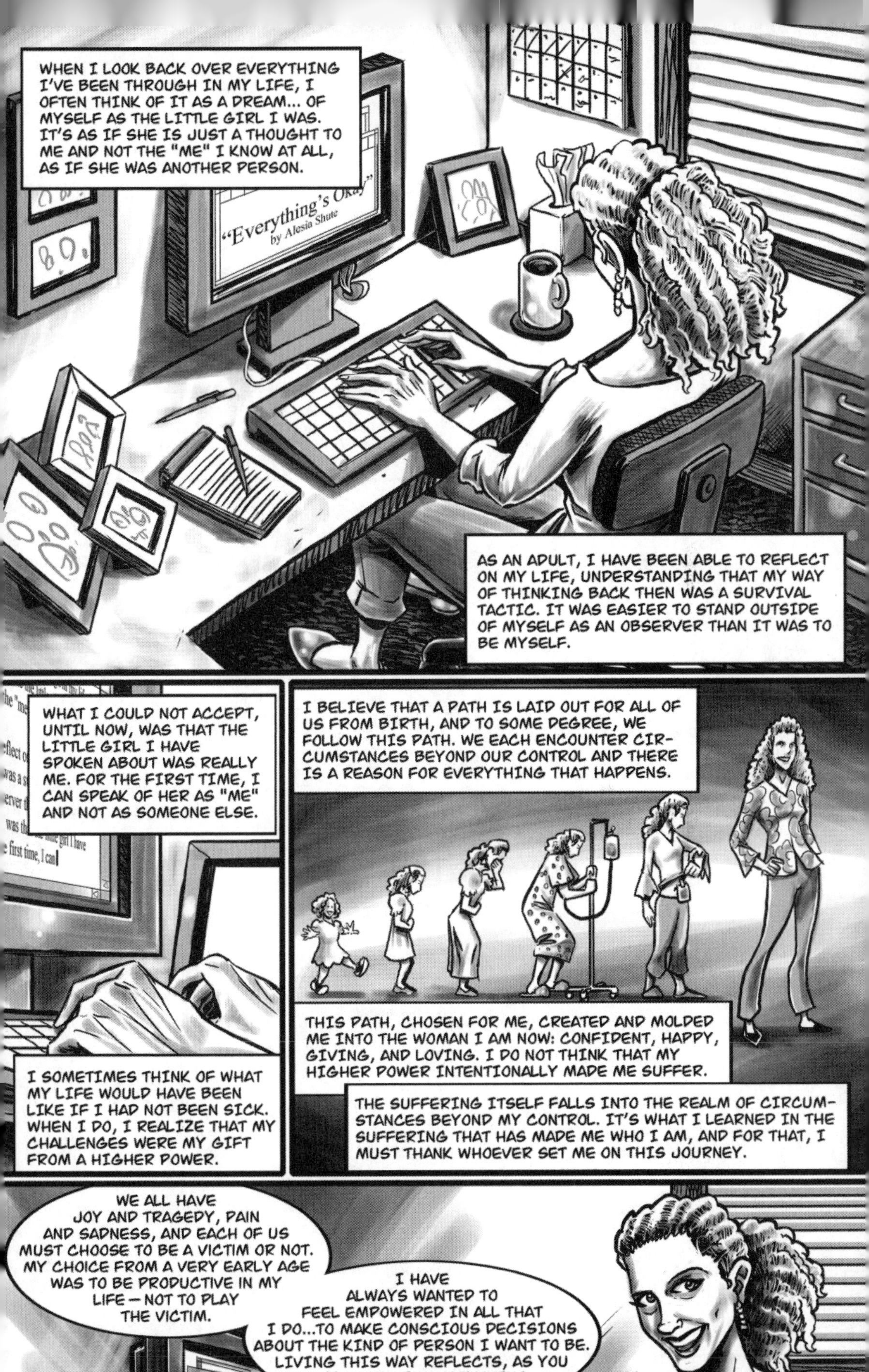
WHEN I LOOK BACK OVER EVERYTHING I'VE BEEN THROUGH IN MY LIFE, I OFTEN THINK OF IT AS A DREAM... OF MYSELF AS THE LITTLE GIRL I WAS. IT'S AS IF SHE IS JUST A THOUGHT TO ME AND NOT THE "ME" I KNOW AT ALL, AS IF SHE WAS ANOTHER PERSON.
"Everything's Okay"
by Alesia Shute
AS AN ADULT, I HAVE BEEN ABLE TO REFLECT ON MY LIFE, UNDERSTANDING THAT MY WAY OF THINKING BACK THEN WAS A SURVIVAL TACTIC. IT WAS EASIER TO STAND OUTSIDE OF MYSELF AS AN OBSERVER THAN IT WAS TO BE MYSELF.
WHAT I COULD NOT ACCEPT, UNTIL NOW, WAS THAT THE LITTLE GIRL I HAVE SPOKEN ABOUT WAS REALLY ME. FOR THE FIRST TIME, I CAN SPEAK OF HER AS "ME" AND NOT AS SOMEONE ELSE.
I SOMETIMES THINK OF WHAT MY LIFE WOULD HAVE BEEN LIKE IF I HAD NOT BEEN SICK. WHEN I DO, I REALIZE THAT MY CHALLENGES WERE MY GIFT FROM A HIGHER POWER.
I BELIEVE THAT A PATH IS LAID OUT FOR ALL OF US FROM BIRTH, AND TO SOME DEGREE, WE FOLLOW THIS PATH. WE EACH ENCOUNTER CIRCUMSTANCES BEYOND OUR CONTROL AND THERE IS A REASON FOR EVERYTHING THAT HAPPENS.
THIS PATH, CHOSEN FOR ME, CREATED AND MOLDED ME INTO THE WOMAN I AM NOW: CONFIDENT, HAPPY, GIVING, AND LOVING. I DO NOT THINK THAT MY HIGHER POWER INTENTIONALLY MADE ME SUFFER.
THE SUFFERING ITSELF FALLS INTO THE REALM OF CIRCUMSTANCES BEYOND MY CONTROL. IT'S WHAT I LEARNED IN THE SUFFERING THAT HAS MADE ME WHO I AM, AND FOR THAT, I MUST THANK WHOEVER SET ME ON THIS JOURNEY.
WE ALL HAVE JOY AND TRAGEDY, PAIN AND SADNESS, AND EACH OF US MUST CHOOSE TO BE A VICTIM OR NOT. MY CHOICE FROM A VERY EARLY AGE WAS TO BE PRODUCTIVE IN MY LIFE — NOT TO PLAY THE VICTIM.
I HAVE ALWAYS WANTED TO FEEL EMPOWERED IN ALL THAT I DO...TO MAKE CONSCIOUS DECISIONS ABOUT THE KIND OF PERSON I WANT TO BE. LIVING THIS WAY REFLECTS, AS YOU WILL SEE, IN EVERYTHING THAT I DO.

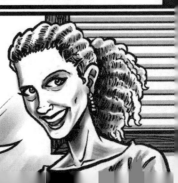

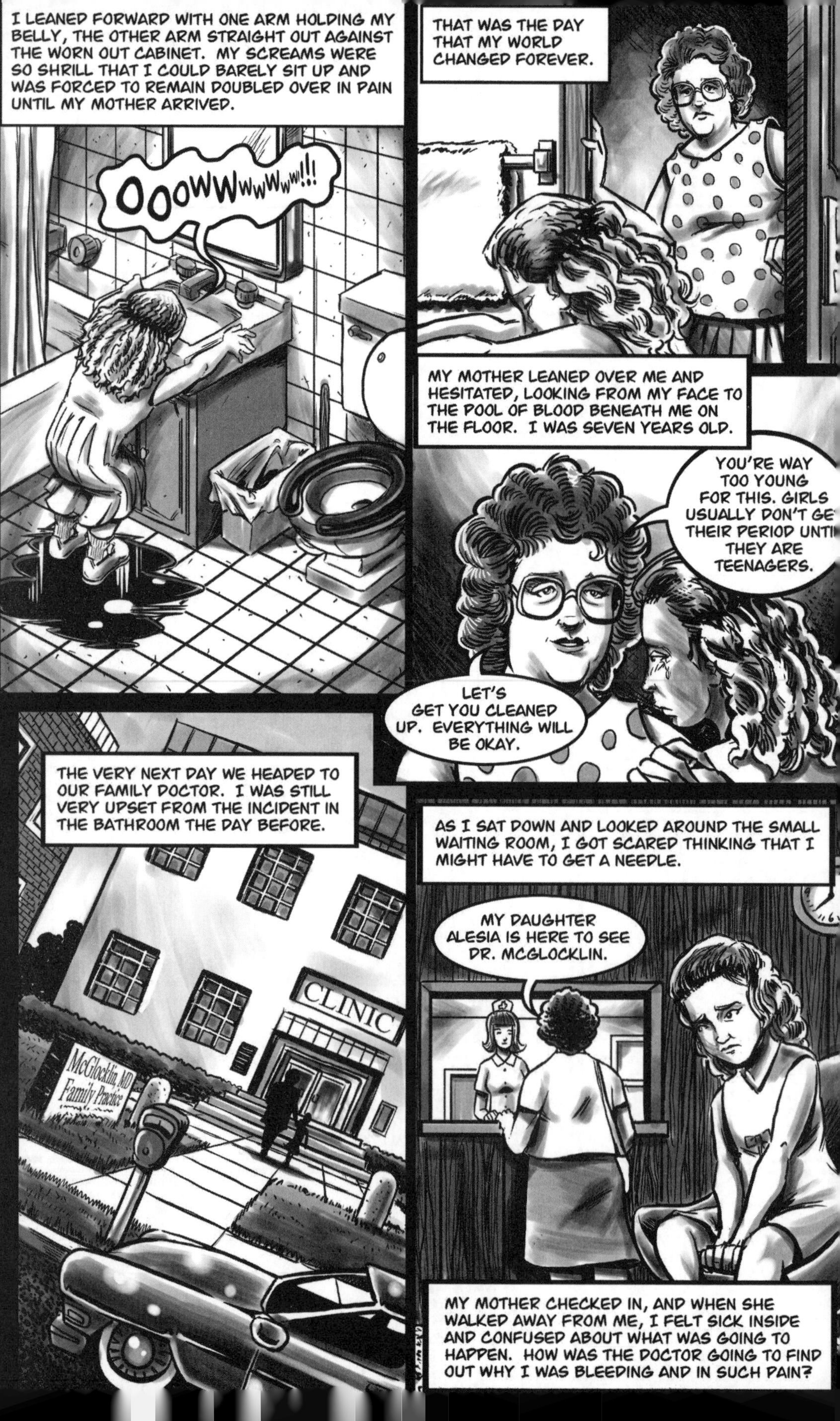
I LEANED FORWARD WITH ONE ARM HOLDING MY BELLY, THE OTHER ARM STRAIGHT OUT AGAINST THE WORN OUT CABINET. MY SCREAMS WERE SO SHRILL THAT I COULD BARELY SIT UP AND WAS FORCED TO REMAIN DOUBLED OVER IN PAIN UNTIL MY MOTHER ARRIVED.
OOOWWwwwwww!!!
THAT WAS THE DAY THAT MY WORLD CHANGED FOREVER.
MY MOTHER LEANED OVER ME AND HESITATED, LOOKING FROM MY FACE TO THE POOL OF BLOOD BENEATH ME ON THE FLOOR. I WAS SEVEN YEARS OLD.
YOU'RE WAY TOO YOUNG FOR THIS. GIRLS USUALLY DON'T GE THEIR PERIOD UNTI THEY ARE TEENAGERS.
LET'S GET YOU CLEANED UP. EVERYTHING WILL BE OKAY.
THE VERY NEXT DAY WE HEADED TO OUR FAMILY DOCTOR. I WAS STILL VERY UPSET FROM THE INCIDENT IN THE BATHROOM THE DAY BEFORE.
CLINIC
McGlocklin, MD Family Practice
AS I SAT DOWN AND LOOKED AROUND THE SMALL WAITING ROOM, I GOT SCARED THINKING THAT I MIGHT HAVE TO GET A NEEDLE.
MY DAUGHTER ALESIA IS HERE TO SEE DR. MCGLOCKLIN.
MY MOTHER CHECKED IN, AND WHEN SHE WALKED AWAY FROM ME, I FELT SICK INSIDE AND CONFUSED ABOUT WHAT WAS GOING TO HAPPEN. HOW WAS THE DOCTOR GOING TO FIND OUT WHY I WAS BLEEDING AND IN SUCH PAIN?

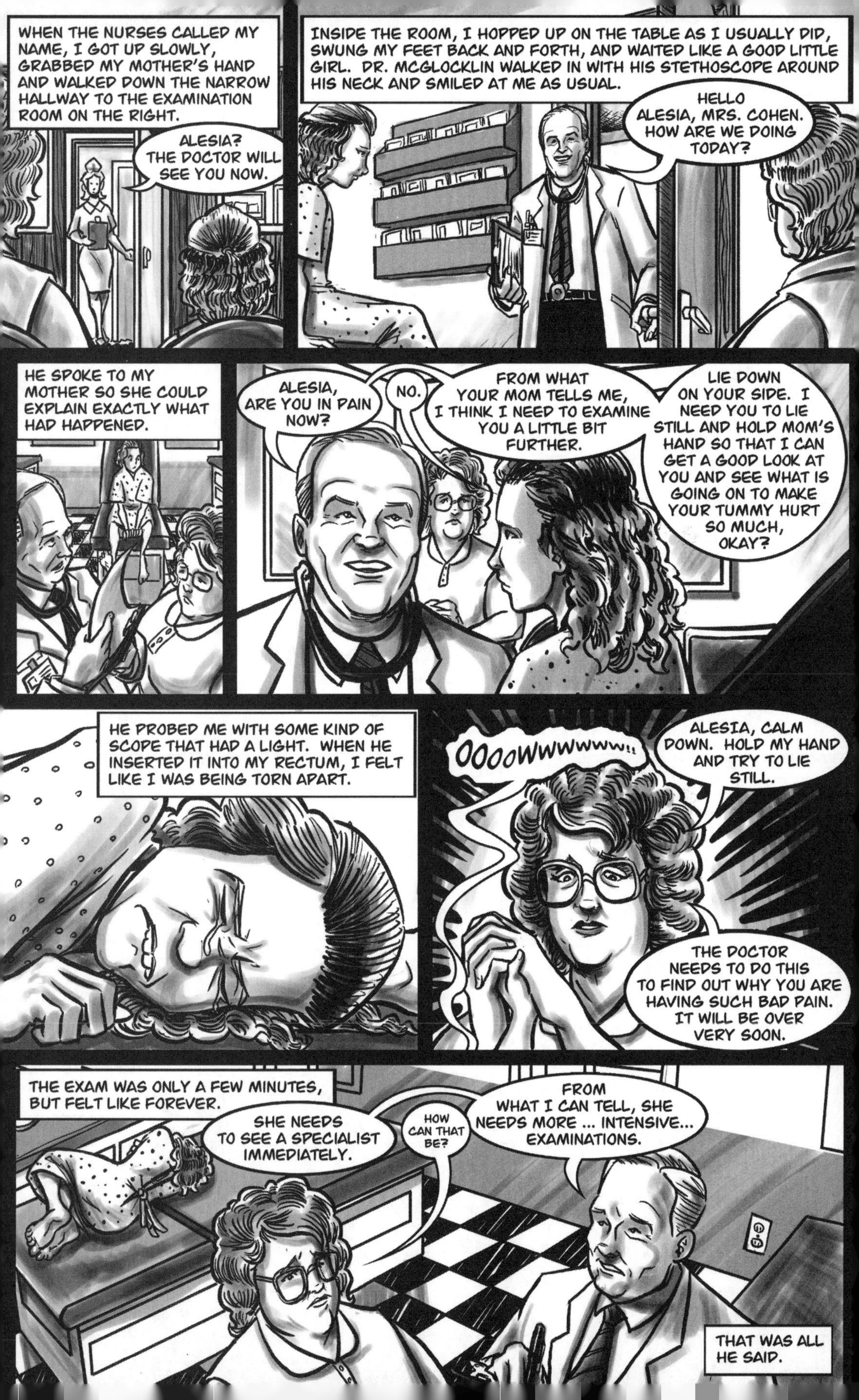
WHEN THE NURSES CALLED MY NAME, I GOT UP SLOWLY, GRABBED MY MOTHER'S HAND AND WALKED DOWN THE NARROW HALLWAY TO THE EXAMINATION ROOM ON THE RIGHT.
ALESIA? THE DOCTOR WILL SEE YOU NOW.
INSIDE THE ROOM, I HOPPED UP ON THE TABLE AS I USUALLY DID, SWUNG MY FEET BACK AND FORTH, AND WAITED LIKE A GOOD LITTLE GIRL. DR. MCGLOCKLIN WALKED IN WITH HIS STETHOSCOPE AROUND HIS NECK AND SMILED AT ME AS USUAL.
HELLO ALESIA, MRS. COHEN. HOW ARE WE DOING TODAY?
HE SPOKE TO MY MOTHER SO SHE COULD EXPLAIN EXACTLY WHAT HAD HAPPENED.
ALESIA, ARE YOU IN PAIN NOW?
NO.
FROM WHAT YOUR MOM TELLS ME, I THINK I NEED TO EXAMINE YOU A LITTLE BIT FURTHER.
LIE DOWN ON YOUR SIDE. I NEED YOU TO LIE STILL AND HOLD MOM'S HAND SO THAT I CAN GET A GOOD LOOK AT YOU AND SEE WHAT IS GOING ON TO MAKE YOUR TUMMY HURT SO MUCH, OKAY?
HE PROBED ME WITH SOME KIND OF SCOPE THAT HAD A LIGHT. WHEN HE INSERTED IT INTO MY RECTUM, I FELT LIKE I WAS BEING TORN APART.
OOOOWWWWWW!!
ALESIA, CALM DOWN. HOLD MY HAND AND TRY TO LIE STILL.
THE DOCTOR NEEDS TO DO THIS TO FIND OUT WHY YOU ARE HAVING SUCH BAD PAIN. IT WILL BE OVER VERY SOON.
THE EXAM WAS ONLY A FEW MINUTES, BUT FELT LIKE FOREVER.
SHE NEEDS TO SEE A SPECIALIST IMMEDIATELY.
HOW CAN THAT BE?
FROM WHAT I CAN TELL, SHE NEEDS MORE ... INTENSIVE... EXAMINATIONS.
THAT WAS ALL HE SAID.

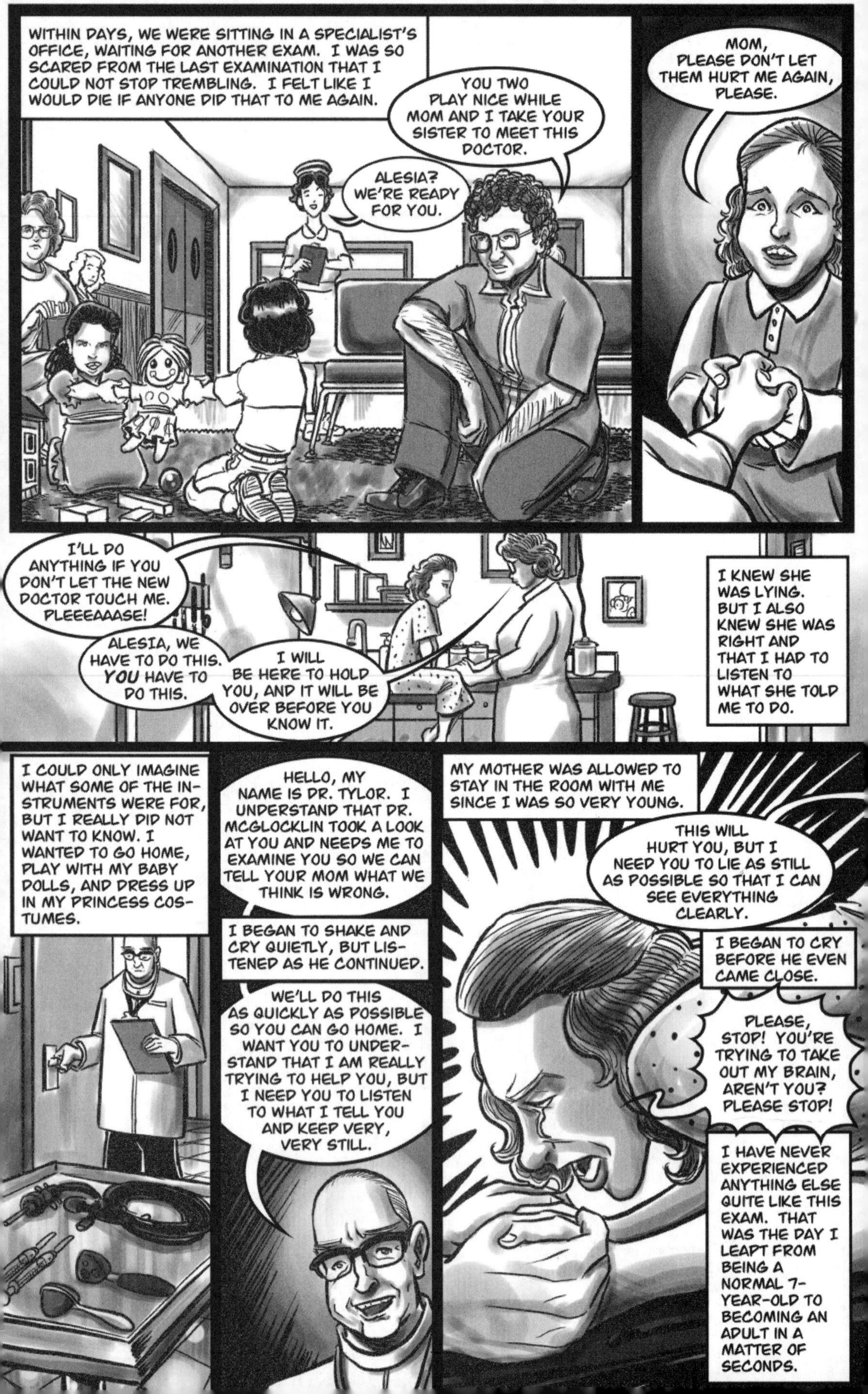

WITHIN DAYS, WE WERE SITTING IN A SPECIALIST'S OFFICE, WAITING FOR ANOTHER EXAM. I WAS SO SCARED FROM THE LAST EXAMINATION THAT I COULD NOT STOP TREMBLING. I FELT LIKE I WOULD DIE IF ANYONE DID THAT TO ME AGAIN.
YOU TWO PLAY NICE WHILE MOM AND I TAKE YOUR SISTER TO MEET THIS DOCTOR.
ALESIA? WE'RE READY FOR YOU.
MOM, PLEASE DON'T LET THEM HURT ME AGAIN, PLEASE.
I'LL DO ANYTHING IF YOU DON'T LET THE NEW DOCTOR TOUCH ME. PLEEEAAASE!
ALESIA, WE HAVE TO DO THIS. YOU HAVE TO DO THIS.
I WILL BE HERE TO HOLD YOU, AND IT WILL BE OVER BEFORE YOU KNOW IT.
I KNEW SHE WAS LYING. BUT I ALSO KNEW SHE WAS RIGHT AND THAT I HAD TO LISTEN TO WHAT SHE TOLD ME TO DO.
I COULD ONLY IMAGINE WHAT SOME OF THE INSTRUMENTS WERE FOR, BUT I REALLY DID NOT WANT TO KNOW. I WANTED TO GO HOME, PLAY WITH MY BABY DOLLS, AND DRESS UP IN MY PRINCESS COSTUMES.
HELLO, MY NAME IS DR. TYLOR. I UNDERSTAND THAT DR. MCGLOCKLIN TOOK A LOOK AT YOU AND NEEDS ME TO EXAMINE YOU SO WE CAN TELL YOUR MOM WHAT WE THINK IS WRONG.
I BEGAN TO SHAKE AND CRY QUIETLY, BUT LISTENED AS HE CONTINUED.
WE'LL DO THIS AS QUICKLY AS POSSIBLE SO YOU CAN GO HOME. I WANT YOU TO UNDERSTAND THAT I AM REALLY TRYING TO HELP YOU, BUT I NEED YOU TO LISTEN TO WHAT I TELL YOU AND KEEP VERY, VERY STILL.
MY MOTHER WAS ALLOWED TO STAY IN THE ROOM WITH ME SINCE I WAS SO VERY YOUNG.
THIS WILL HURT YOU, BUT I NEED YOU TO LIE AS STILL AS POSSIBLE SO THAT I CAN SEE EVERYTHING CLEARLY.
I BEGAN TO CRY BEFORE HE EVEN CAME CLOSE.
PLEASE, STOP! YOU'RE TRYING TO TAKE OUT MY BRAIN, AREN'T YOU? PLEASE STOP!
I HAVE NEVER EXPERIENCED ANYTHING ELSE QUITE LIKE THIS EXAM. THAT WAS THE DAY I LEAPT FROM BEING A NORMAL 7-YEAR-OLD TO BECOMING AN ADULT IN A MATTER OF SECONDS.

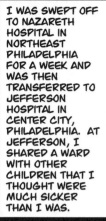

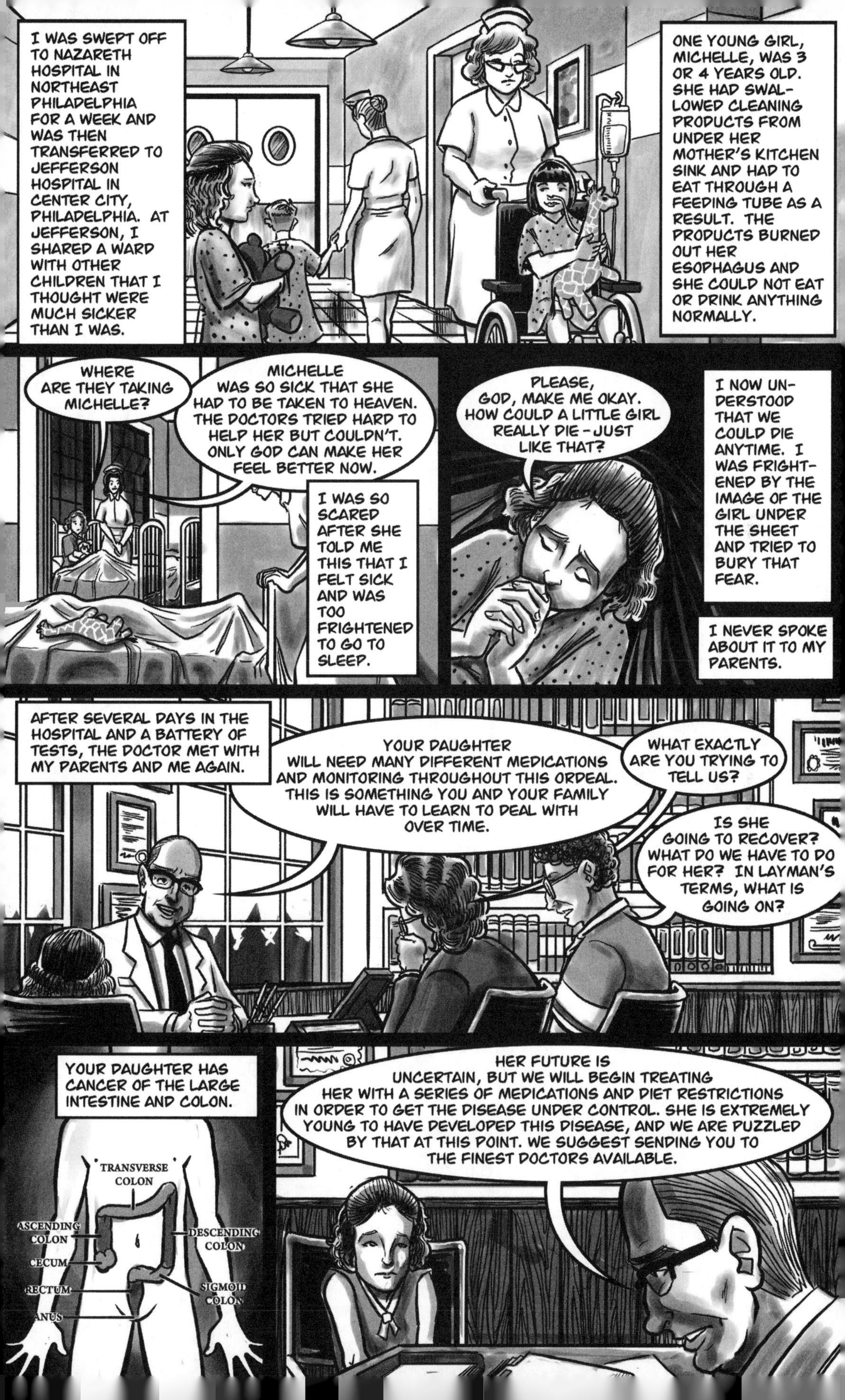

I WAS SWEPT OFF TO NAZARETH HOSPITAL IN NORTHEAST PHILADELPHIA FOR A WEEK AND WAS THEN TRANSFERRED TO JEFFERSON HOSPITAL IN CENTER CITY, PHILADELPHIA. AT JEFFERSON, I SHARED A WARD WITH OTHER CHILDREN THAT I THOUGHT WERE MUCH SICKER THAN I WAS.

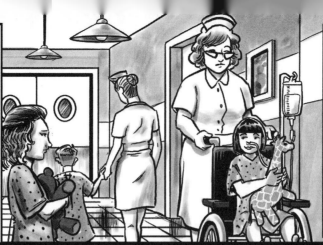

ONE YOUNG GIRL, MICHELLE, WAS 3 OR 4 YEARS OLD. SHE HAD SWALLOWED CLEANING PRODUCTS FROM UNDER HER MOTHER'S KITCHEN SINK AND HAD TO EAT THROUGH A FEEDING TUBE AS A RESULT. THE PRODUCTS BURNED OUT HER ESOPHAGUS AND SHE COULD NOT EAT OR DRINK ANYTHING NORMALLY.

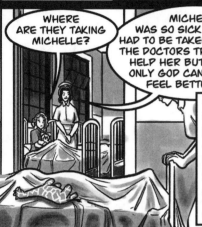

WHERE ARE THEY TAKING MICHELLE?

MICHELLE WAS SO SICK THAT SHE HAD TO BE TAKEN TO HEAVEN. THE DOCTORS TRIED HARD TO HELP HER BUT COULDN'T. ONLY GOD CAN MAKE HER FEEL BETTER NOW.

I WAS SO SCARED AFTER SHE TOLD ME THIS THAT I FELT SICK AND WAS TOO FRIGHTENED TO GO TO SLEEP.

PLEASE, GOD, MAKE ME OKAY. HOW COULD A LITTLE GIRL REALLY DIE – JUST LIKE THAT?

I NOW UNDERSTOOD THAT WE COULD DIE ANYTIME. I WAS FRIGHTENED BY THE IMAGE OF THE GIRL UNDER THE SHEET AND TRIED TO BURY THAT FEAR.

I NEVER SPOKE ABOUT IT TO MY PARENTS.

AFTER SEVERAL DAYS IN THE HOSPITAL AND A BATTERY OF TESTS, THE DOCTOR MET WITH MY PARENTS AND ME AGAIN.

YOUR DAUGHTER WILL NEED MANY DIFFERENT MEDICATIONS AND MONITORING THROUGHOUT THIS ORDEAL. THIS IS SOMETHING YOU AND YOUR FAMILY WILL HAVE TO LEARN TO DEAL WITH OVER TIME.

WHAT EXACTLY ARE YOU TRYING TO TELL US?

IS SHE GOING TO RECOVER? WHAT DO WE HAVE TO DO FOR HER? IN LAYMAN'S TERMS, WHAT IS GOING ON?

YOUR DAUGHTER HAS CANCER OF THE LARGE INTESTINE AND COLON.

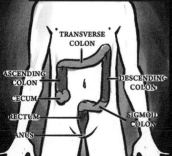

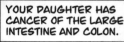

TRANSVERSE COLON

ASCENDING COLON

CECUM

RECTUM

DESCENDING COLON

SIGMOID COLON

ANUS

HER FUTURE IS UNCERTAIN, BUT WE WILL BEGIN TREATING HER WITH A SERIES OF MEDICATIONS AND DIET RESTRICTIONS IN ORDER TO GET THE DISEASE UNDER CONTROL. SHE IS EXTREMELY YOUNG TO HAVE DEVELOPED THIS DISEASE, AND WE ARE PUZZLED BY THAT AT THIS POINT. WE SUGGEST SENDING YOU TO THE FINEST DOCTORS AVAILABLE.

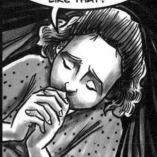

I STARTED TO DETACH MYSELF FROM THE PAIN... A SURVIVAL TECHNIQUE. THE PAIN BECAME A PART OF LIFE. FOR THE NEXT FEW YEARS, UNTIL I WAS ABOUT TEN, I SPENT MORE TIME IN HOSPITALS THAN OUT.

WITHOUT ANY OF US REALIZING IT, ALL OF OUR LIVES BEGAN TO CHANGE. EVERY PLAN FOR EVERY DAY WOULD DANGLE RELATIVE TO HOW SICK OR WEAK I WAS, OR HOW MANY APPOINTMENTS I HAD. WE ALL BECAME SICK— NOT JUST ME.

THE LEVEL OF MATURITY I REACHED BY AGE 10 WAS STAGGERING. THOSE WERE THE CARDS I WAS DEALT. I BEGAN TO LOOK AT MYSELF AS ONE PERSON AND AT THE SICK CHILD AS SOMEONE ELSE.

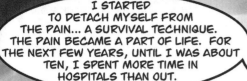
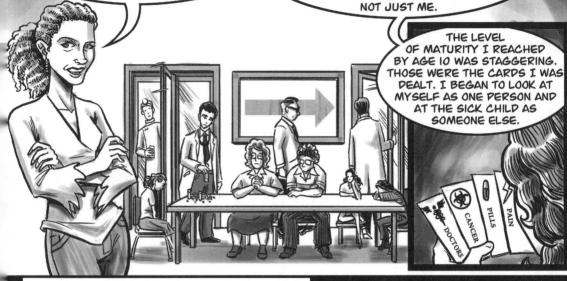

DOCTORS
CANCER
PILLS
PAIN

WHEN I WAS HOME FROM THE HOSPITAL, MY LIFE WAS ANYTHING BUT WHAT I TRULY WANTED. I AWOKE EVERY MORNING TO BREAKFAST AND DOZENS OF PILLS. I WOULD CRY THROUGH EVERY SWALLOW. I DO NOT EVEN KNOW HOW MANY I TOOK DAILY, BUT IT SEEMED LIKE PILES.

TRY TO EAT SOMETHING AND TAKE YOUR PILLS.

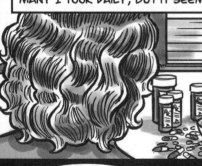

DO I HAVE TO? WHY DO I HAVE TO DO THIS?

THEN LUNCHTIME WOULD COME WITH THE SAME RITUAL, AS WOULD DINNER.

IS THAT THE PILL THAT'S GOING TO MAKE YOU SMELL BETTER?

I BET THERE ISN'T ONE STRONG ENOUGH.

MAYBE IT'LL TURN YOUR SKIN PURPLE!

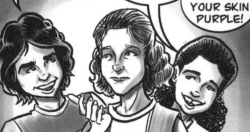

AFTER EACH MEAL, WHEN EVERYONE WAS DONE AND MOM WAS DOING THE DISHES, I WAS STILL SITTING THERE, NOT WANTING TO EAT AND NOT WANTING TO TAKE THE PILLS. MY DAD WOULD SIT WITH ME AND COAX ME TO FINISH, SOMETIMES INTO THE EVENING.

MY SISTER AND BROTHER WOULD MAKE FUN OF ME BECAUSE I HAD SO MUCH MEDICINE TO TAKE. WE WERE NORMAL SIBLINGS, TAUNTING EACH OTHER, BUT THEY HAD MORE STUFF TO TAUNT ME WITH.

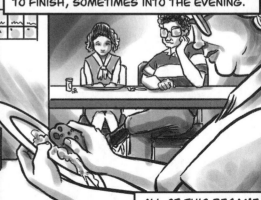

ALL OF THIS BECAME OUR ROUTINE.

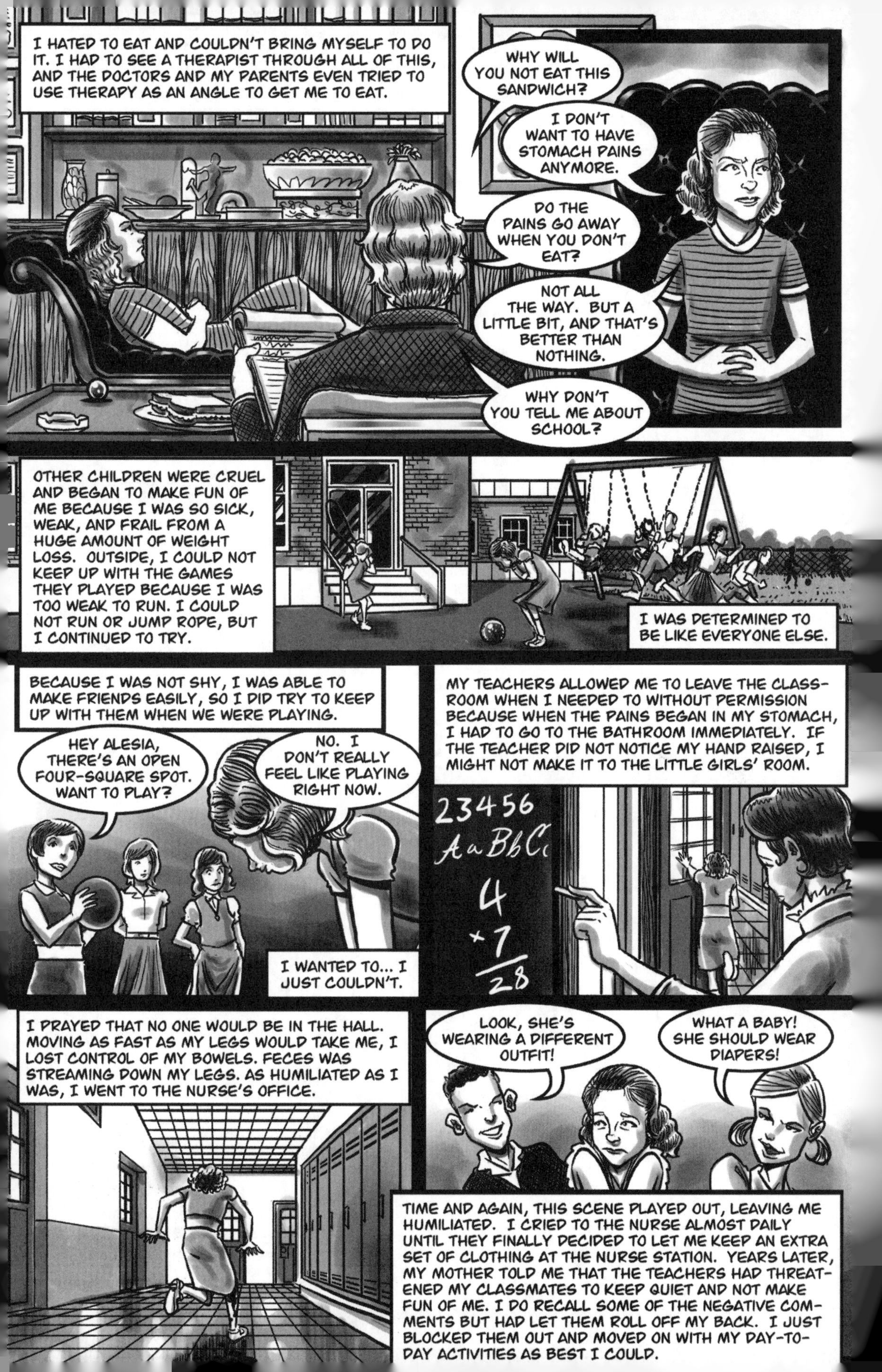
I HATED TO EAT AND COULDN'T BRING MYSELF TO DO IT. I HAD TO SEE A THERAPIST THROUGH ALL OF THIS, AND THE DOCTORS AND MY PARENTS EVEN TRIED TO USE THERAPY AS AN ANGLE TO GET ME TO EAT.
WHY WILL YOU NOT EAT THIS SANDWICH?
I DON'T WANT TO HAVE STOMACH PAINS ANYMORE.
DO THE PAINS GO AWAY WHEN YOU DON'T EAT?
NOT ALL THE WAY. BUT A LITTLE BIT, AND THAT'S BETTER THAN NOTHING.
WHY DON'T YOU TELL ME ABOUT SCHOOL?
OTHER CHILDREN WERE CRUEL AND BEGAN TO MAKE FUN OF ME BECAUSE I WAS SO SICK, WEAK, AND FRAIL FROM A HUGE AMOUNT OF WEIGHT LOSS. OUTSIDE, I COULD NOT KEEP UP WITH THE GAMES THEY PLAYED BECAUSE I WAS TOO WEAK TO RUN. I COULD NOT RUN OR JUMP ROPE, BUT I CONTINUED TO TRY.
I WAS DETERMINED TO BE LIKE EVERYONE ELSE.
BECAUSE I WAS NOT SHY, I WAS ABLE TO MAKE FRIENDS EASILY, SO I DID TRY TO KEEP UP WITH THEM WHEN WE WERE PLAYING.
HEY ALESIA, THERE'S AN OPEN FOUR-SQUARE SPOT. WANT TO PLAY?
NO. I DON'T REALLY FEEL LIKE PLAYING RIGHT NOW.
I WANTED TO... I JUST COULDN'T.
MY TEACHERS ALLOWED ME TO LEAVE THE CLASS-ROOM WHEN I NEEDED TO WITHOUT PERMISSION BECAUSE WHEN THE PAINS BEGAN IN MY STOMACH, I HAD TO GO TO THE BATHROOM IMMEDIATELY. IF THE TEACHER DID NOT NOTICE MY HAND RAISED, I MIGHT NOT MAKE IT TO THE LITTLE GIRLS' ROOM.
23456
Aa Bb Cc
4
×7
28
I PRAYED THAT NO ONE WOULD BE IN THE HALL. MOVING AS FAST AS MY LEGS WOULD TAKE ME, I LOST CONTROL OF MY BOWELS. FECES WAS STREAMING DOWN MY LEGS. AS HUMILIATED AS I WAS, I WENT TO THE NURSE'S OFFICE.
LOOK, SHE'S WEARING A DIFFERENT OUTFIT!
WHAT A BABY! SHE SHOULD WEAR DIAPERS!
TIME AND AGAIN, THIS SCENE PLAYED OUT, LEAVING ME HUMILIATED. I CRIED TO THE NURSE ALMOST DAILY UNTIL THEY FINALLY DECIDED TO LET ME KEEP AN EXTRA SET OF CLOTHING AT THE NURSE STATION. YEARS LATER, MY MOTHER TOLD ME THAT THE TEACHERS HAD THREAT-ENED MY CLASSMATES TO KEEP QUIET AND NOT MAKE FUN OF ME. I DO RECALL SOME OF THE NEGATIVE COM-MENTS BUT HAD LET THEM ROLL OFF MY BACK. I JUST BLOCKED THEM OUT AND MOVED ON WITH MY DAY-TO-DAY ACTIVITIES AS BEST I COULD.

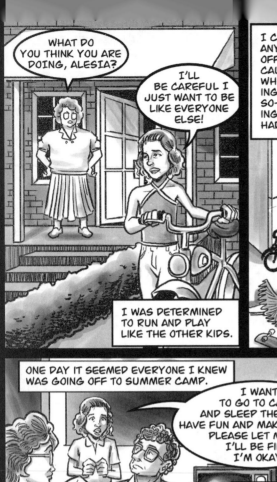

WHAT DO YOU THINK YOU ARE DOING, ALESIA?

I'LL BE CAREFUL I JUST WANT TO BE LIKE EVERYONE ELSE!

I WAS DETERMINED TO PLAY AND RUN LIKE THE OTHER KIDS.

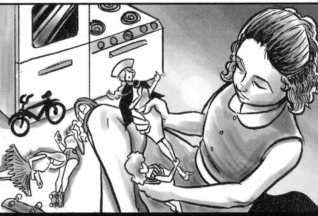

I CONSIDERED MYSELF NON-ATHLETIC. I DIDN'T PLAY ANY SPORTS IN SCHOOL, PARTLY BECAUSE THEY WEREN'T OFFERED TO GIRLS IN THE LATE 1960S AND PARTLY BECAUSE I SIMPLY WASN'T VERY INTERESTED. TRUTH WAS, WHILE PART OF ME FELT LIKE I SHOULD BE ROLLER-SKATING, BIKE RIDING, AND SKATEBOARDING, I PREFERRED SO-CALLED "GIRLY THINGS," AND IT PROBABLY HAD NOTHING TO DO WITH MY ILLNESS. STILL, PART OF ME FELT I HAD TO LIVE UP TO MY FRIENDS' EXPECTATIONS.

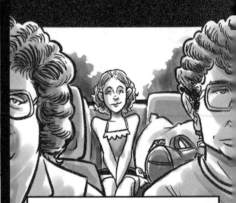

ONE DAY IT SEEMED EVERYONE I KNEW WAS GOING OFF TO SUMMER CAMP.

I WANT TO GO TO CAMP AND SLEEP THERE AND HAVE FUN AND MAKE FRIENDS! PLEASE LET ME GO! I'LL BE FINE! I'M OKAY!

GOING TO OVER-NIGHT CAMP LIKE MY BIG BROTHER WAS SO IMPORTANT TO ME, AND, ALTHOUGH I WAS A BIT YOUNG, THEY FINALLY GAVE IN.

THE RIDE WAS SO EXCITING THAT I BARELY REALIZED IT WAS NEARLY THREE HOURS LONG.

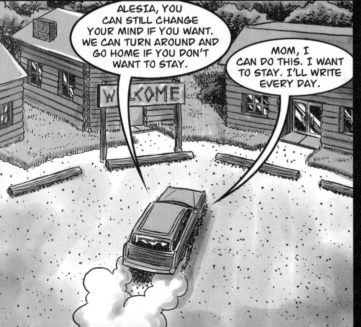

ALESIA, YOU CAN STILL CHANGE YOUR MIND IF YOU WANT. WE CAN TURN AROUND AND GO HOME IF YOU DON'T WANT TO STAY.

MOM, I CAN DO THIS. I WANT TO STAY. I'LL WRITE EVERY DAY.

WELCOME

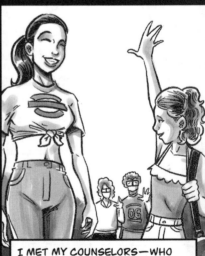

I MET MY COUNSELORS—WHO TURNED OUT TO BE A GROUP OF TEENAGE GIRLS—AND INSTANTLY FELL IN LOVE WITH THEM. THEY WERE GREAT TO ME AND SEEMED COOL AND EASY TO GET TO KNOW.

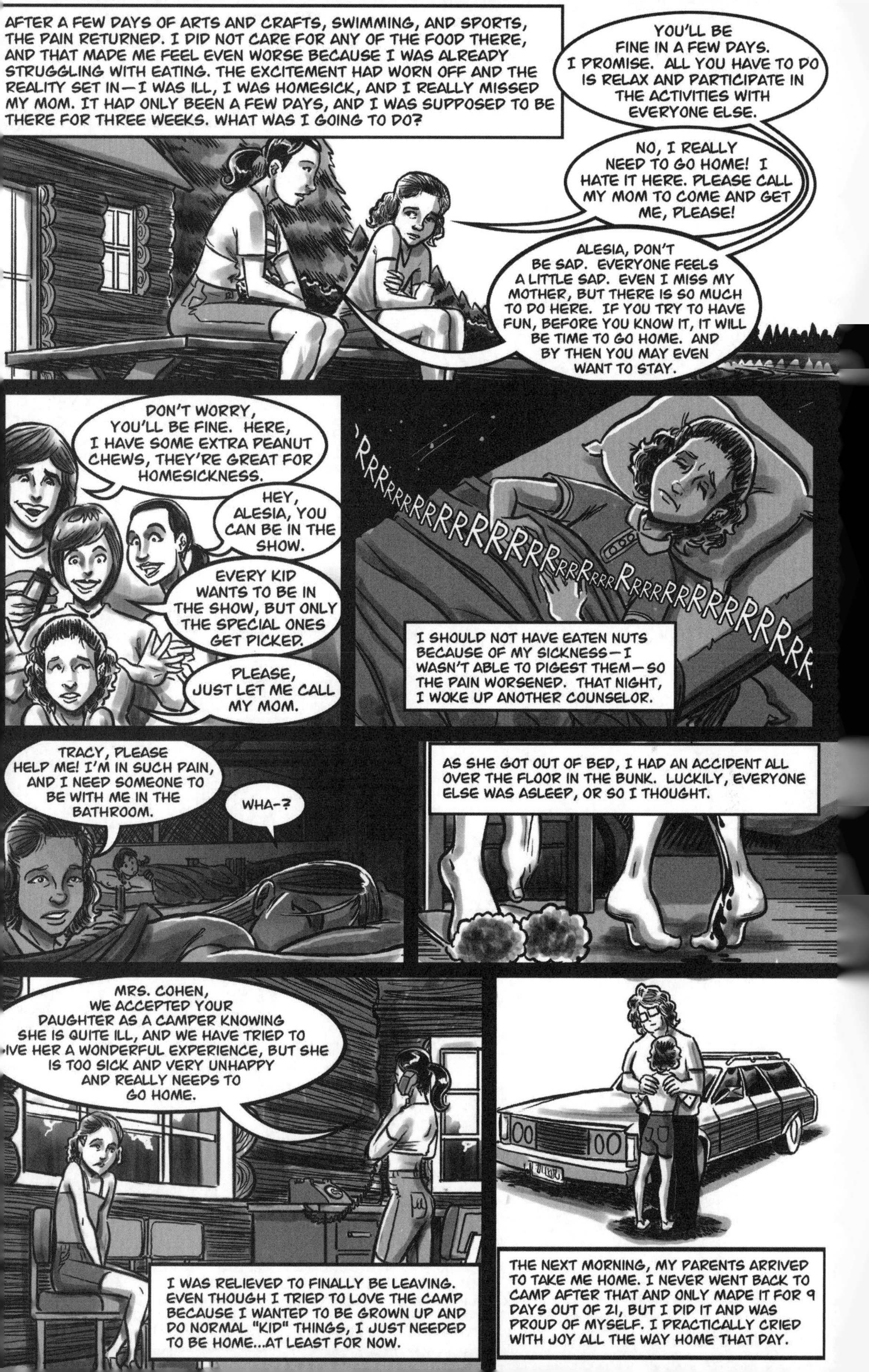
AFTER A FEW DAYS OF ARTS AND CRAFTS, SWIMMING, AND SPORTS, THE PAIN RETURNED. I DID NOT CARE FOR ANY OF THE FOOD THERE, AND THAT MADE ME FEEL EVEN WORSE BECAUSE I WAS ALREADY STRUGGLING WITH EATING. THE EXCITEMENT HAD WORN OFF AND THE REALITY SET IN—I WAS ILL, I WAS HOMESICK, AND I REALLY MISSED MY MOM. IT HAD ONLY BEEN A FEW DAYS, AND I WAS SUPPOSED TO BE THERE FOR THREE WEEKS. WHAT WAS I GOING TO DO?
YOU'LL BE FINE IN A FEW DAYS. I PROMISE. ALL YOU HAVE TO DO IS RELAX AND PARTICIPATE IN THE ACTIVITIES WITH EVERYONE ELSE.
NO, I REALLY NEED TO GO HOME! I HATE IT HERE. PLEASE CALL MY MOM TO COME AND GET ME, PLEASE!
ALESIA, DON'T BE SAD. EVERYONE FEELS A LITTLE SAD. EVEN I MISS MY MOTHER, BUT THERE IS SO MUCH TO DO HERE. IF YOU TRY TO HAVE FUN, BEFORE YOU KNOW IT, IT WILL BE TIME TO GO HOME. AND BY THEN YOU MAY EVEN WANT TO STAY.
DON'T WORRY, YOU'LL BE FINE. HERE, I HAVE SOME EXTRA PEANUT CHEWS, THEY'RE GREAT FOR HOMESICKNESS.
HEY, ALESIA, YOU CAN BE IN THE SHOW.
EVERY KID WANTS TO BE IN THE SHOW, BUT ONLY THE SPECIAL ONES GET PICKED.
PLEASE, JUST LET ME CALL MY MOM.
'RRRRRRRRRRRRRRRRRRRRRRRRRRRRRRRRRRRRRRR
I SHOULD NOT HAVE EATEN NUTS BECAUSE OF MY SICKNESS—I WASN'T ABLE TO DIGEST THEM—SO THE PAIN WORSENED. THAT NIGHT, I WOKE UP ANOTHER COUNSELOR.
TRACY, PLEASE HELP ME! I'M IN SUCH PAIN, AND I NEED SOMEONE TO BE WITH ME IN THE BATHROOM.
WHA-?
AS SHE GOT OUT OF BED, I HAD AN ACCIDENT ALL OVER THE FLOOR IN THE BUNK. LUCKILY, EVERYONE ELSE WAS ASLEEP, OR SO I THOUGHT.
MRS. COHEN, WE ACCEPTED YOUR DAUGHTER AS A CAMPER KNOWING SHE IS QUITE ILL, AND WE HAVE TRIED TO IVE HER A WONDERFUL EXPERIENCE, BUT SHE IS TOO SICK AND VERY UNHAPPY AND REALLY NEEDS TO GO HOME.
I WAS RELIEVED TO FINALLY BE LEAVING. EVEN THOUGH I TRIED TO LOVE THE CAMP BECAUSE I WANTED TO BE GROWN UP AND DO NORMAL "KID" THINGS, I JUST NEEDED TO BE HOME...AT LEAST FOR NOW.
THE NEXT MORNING, MY PARENTS ARRIVED TO TAKE ME HOME. I NEVER WENT BACK TO CAMP AFTER THAT AND ONLY MADE IT FOR 9 DAYS OUT OF 21, BUT I DID IT AND WAS PROUD OF MYSELF. I PRACTICALLY CRIED WITH JOY ALL THE WAY HOME THAT DAY.

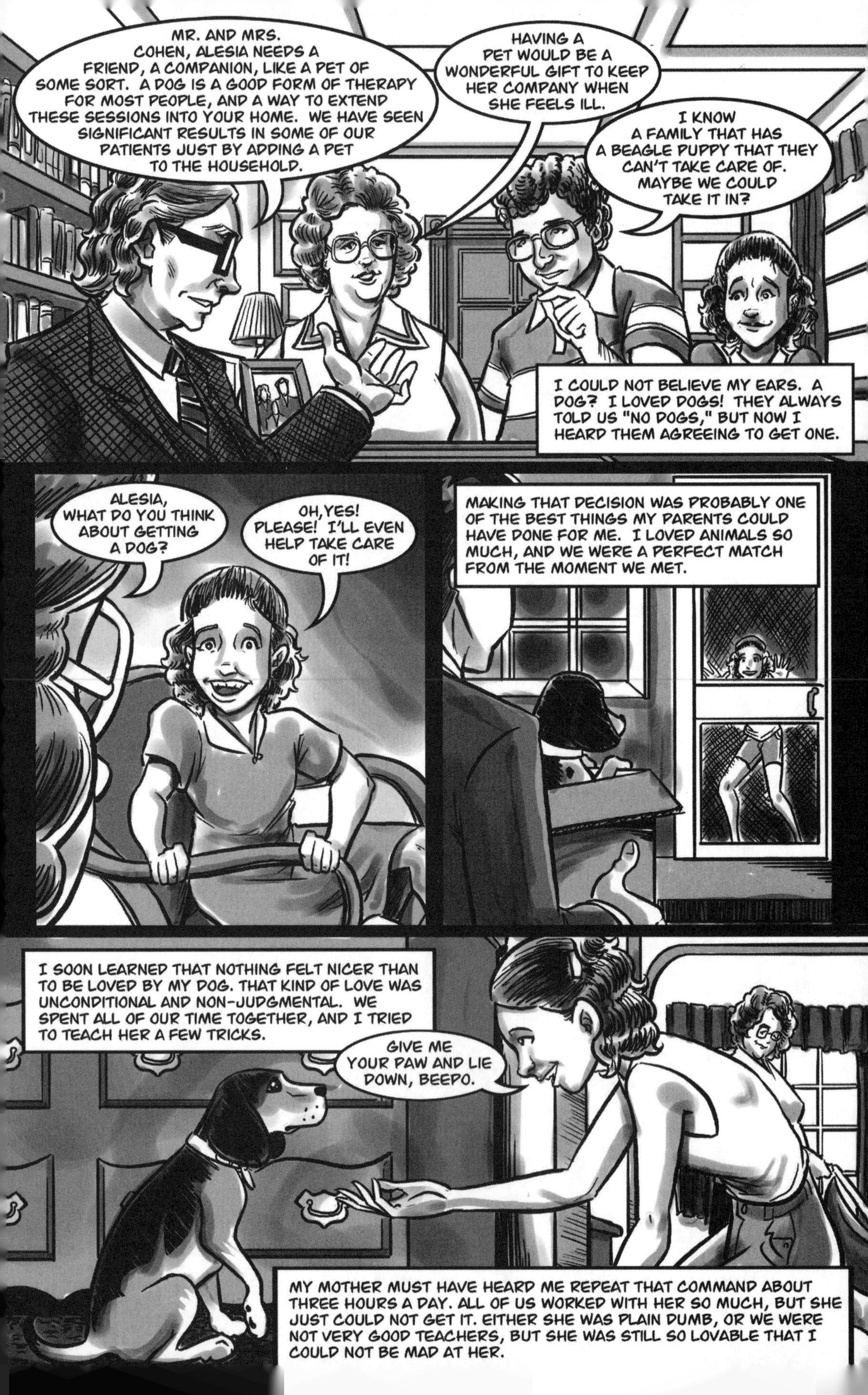
MR. AND MRS. COHEN, ALESIA NEEDS A FRIEND, A COMPANION, LIKE A PET OF SOME SORT. A DOG IS A GOOD FORM OF THERAPY FOR MOST PEOPLE, AND A WAY TO EXTEND THESE SESSIONS INTO YOUR HOME. WE HAVE SEEN SIGNIFICANT RESULTS IN SOME OF OUR PATIENTS JUST BY ADDING A PET TO THE HOUSEHOLD.
HAVING A PET WOULD BE A WONDERFUL GIFT TO KEEP HER COMPANY WHEN SHE FEELS ILL.
I KNOW A FAMILY THAT HAS A BEAGLE PUPPY THAT THEY CAN'T TAKE CARE OF. MAYBE WE COULD TAKE IT IN?
I COULD NOT BELIEVE MY EARS. A DOG? I LOVED DOGS! THEY ALWAYS TOLD US "NO DOGS," BUT NOW I HEARD THEM AGREEING TO GET ONE.
ALESIA, WHAT DO YOU THINK ABOUT GETTING A DOG?
OH, YES! PLEASE! I'LL EVEN HELP TAKE CARE OF IT!
MAKING THAT DECISION WAS PROBABLY ONE OF THE BEST THINGS MY PARENTS COULD HAVE DONE FOR ME. I LOVED ANIMALS SO MUCH, AND WE WERE A PERFECT MATCH FROM THE MOMENT WE MET.
I SOON LEARNED THAT NOTHING FELT NICER THAN TO BE LOVED BY MY DOG. THAT KIND OF LOVE WAS UNCONDITIONAL AND NON-JUDGMENTAL. WE SPENT ALL OF OUR TIME TOGETHER, AND I TRIED TO TEACH HER A FEW TRICKS.
GIVE ME YOUR PAW AND LIE DOWN, BEEPO.
MY MOTHER MUST HAVE HEARD ME REPEAT THAT COMMAND ABOUT THREE HOURS A DAY. ALL OF US WORKED WITH HER SO MUCH, BUT SHE JUST COULD NOT GET IT. EITHER SHE WAS PLAIN DUMB, OR WE WERE NOT VERY GOOD TEACHERS, BUT SHE WAS STILL SO LOVABLE THAT I COULD NOT BE MAD AT HER.

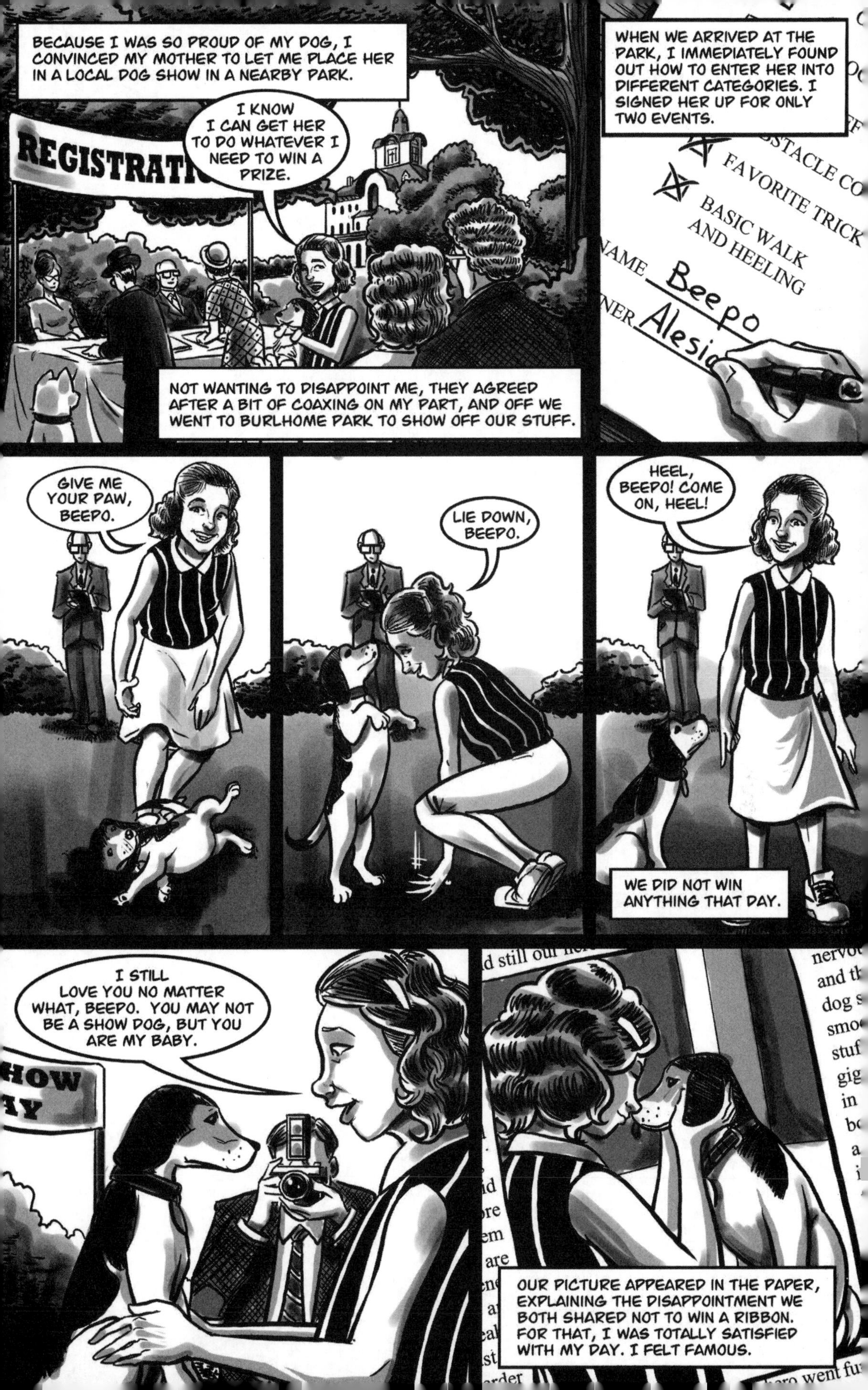
BECAUSE I WAS SO PROUD OF MY DOG, I CONVINCED MY MOTHER TO LET ME PLACE HER IN A LOCAL DOG SHOW IN A NEARBY PARK.
REGISTRATIO
I KNOW I CAN GET HER TO DO WHATEVER I NEED TO WIN A PRIZE.
NOT WANTING TO DISAPPOINT ME, THEY AGREED AFTER A BIT OF COAXING ON MY PART, AND OFF WE WENT TO BURLHOME PARK TO SHOW OFF OUR STUFF.
WHEN WE ARRIVED AT THE PARK, I IMMEDIATELY FOUND OUT HOW TO ENTER HER INTO DIFFERENT CATEGORIES. I SIGNED HER UP FOR ONLY TWO EVENTS.
STACLE CO
FAVORITE TRICK
BASIC WALK AND HEELING
NAME Beepo
NER Alesia
GIVE ME YOUR PAW, BEEPO.
LIE DOWN, BEEPO.
HEEL, BEEPO! COME ON, HEEL!
WE DID NOT WIN ANYTHING THAT DAY.
I STILL LOVE YOU NO MATTER WHAT, BEEPO. YOU MAY NOT BE A SHOW DOG, BUT YOU ARE MY BABY.
HOW
d still our he
OUR PICTURE APPEARED IN THE PAPER, EXPLAINING THE DISAPPOINTMENT WE BOTH SHARED NOT TO WIN A RIBBON. FOR THAT, I WAS TOTALLY SATISFIED WITH MY DAY. I FELT FAMOUS.
hero went fu

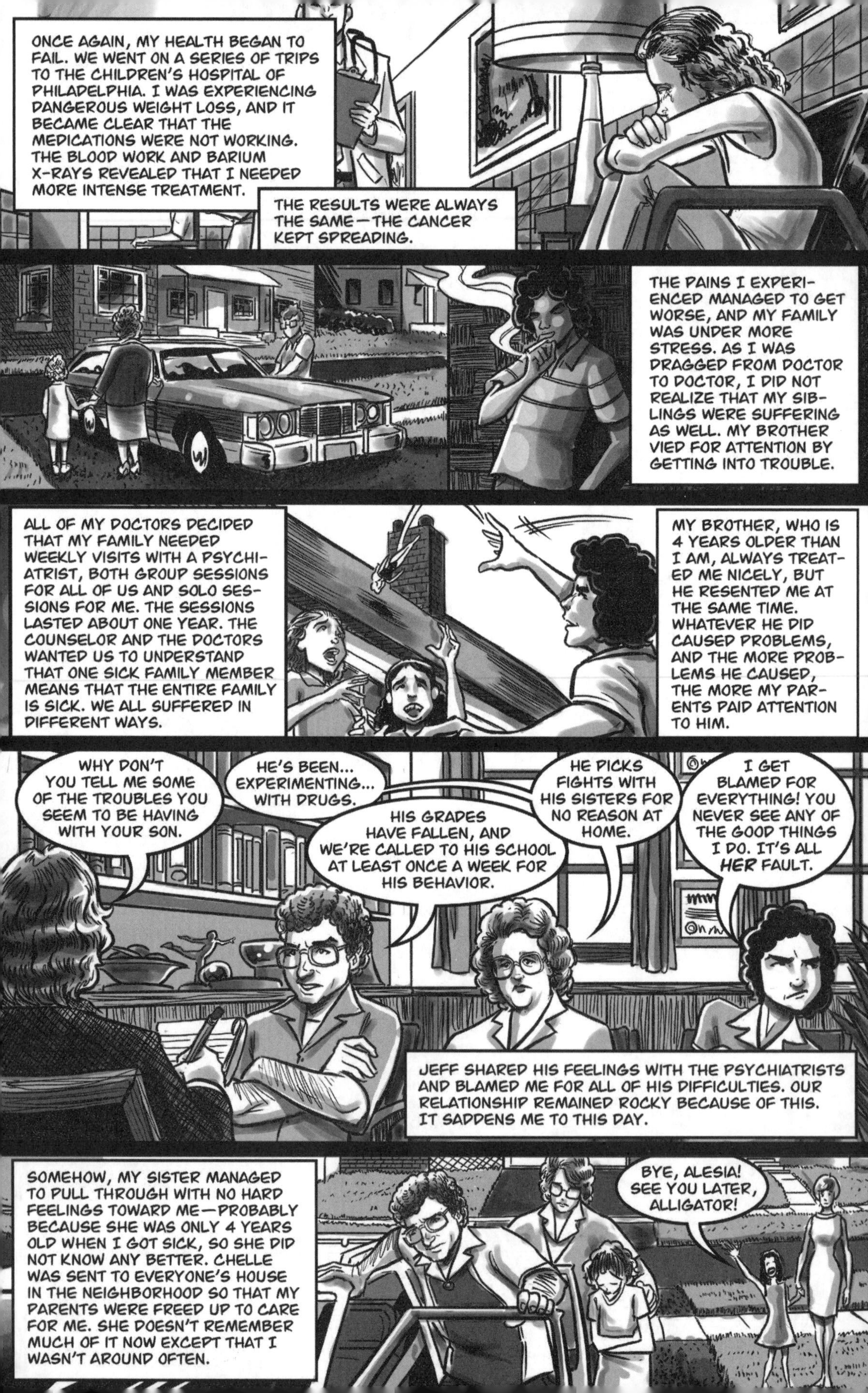
ONCE AGAIN, MY HEALTH BEGAN TO FAIL. WE WENT ON A SERIES OF TRIPS TO THE CHILDREN'S HOSPITAL OF PHILADELPHIA. I WAS EXPERIENCING DANGEROUS WEIGHT LOSS, AND IT BECAME CLEAR THAT THE MEDICATIONS WERE NOT WORKING. THE BLOOD WORK AND BARIUM X-RAYS REVEALED THAT I NEEDED MORE INTENSE TREATMENT.
THE RESULTS WERE ALWAYS THE SAME—THE CANCER KEPT SPREADING.
THE PAINS I EXPERIENCED MANAGED TO GET WORSE, AND MY FAMILY WAS UNDER MORE STRESS. AS I WAS DRAGGED FROM DOCTOR TO DOCTOR, I DID NOT REALIZE THAT MY SIBLINGS WERE SUFFERING AS WELL. MY BROTHER VIED FOR ATTENTION BY GETTING INTO TROUBLE.
ALL OF MY DOCTORS DECIDED THAT MY FAMILY NEEDED WEEKLY VISITS WITH A PSYCHIATRIST, BOTH GROUP SESSIONS FOR ALL OF US AND SOLO SESSIONS FOR ME. THE SESSIONS LASTED ABOUT ONE YEAR. THE COUNSELOR AND THE DOCTORS WANTED US TO UNDERSTAND THAT ONE SICK FAMILY MEMBER MEANS THAT THE ENTIRE FAMILY IS SICK. WE ALL SUFFERED IN DIFFERENT WAYS.
MY BROTHER, WHO IS 4 YEARS OLDER THAN I AM, ALWAYS TREATED ME NICELY, BUT HE RESENTED ME AT THE SAME TIME. WHATEVER HE DID CAUSED PROBLEMS, AND THE MORE PROBLEMS HE CAUSED, THE MORE MY PARENTS PAID ATTENTION TO HIM.
WHY DON'T YOU TELL ME SOME OF THE TROUBLES YOU SEEM TO BE HAVING WITH YOUR SON.
HE'S BEEN... EXPERIMENTING... WITH DRUGS.
HIS GRADES HAVE FALLEN, AND WE'RE CALLED TO HIS SCHOOL AT LEAST ONCE A WEEK FOR HIS BEHAVIOR.
HE PICKS FIGHTS WITH HIS SISTERS FOR NO REASON AT HOME.
I GET BLAMED FOR EVERYTHING! YOU NEVER SEE ANY OF THE GOOD THINGS I DO. IT'S ALL HER FAULT.
JEFF SHARED HIS FEELINGS WITH THE PSYCHIATRISTS AND BLAMED ME FOR ALL OF HIS DIFFICULTIES. OUR RELATIONSHIP REMAINED ROCKY BECAUSE OF THIS. IT SADDENS ME TO THIS DAY.
SOMEHOW, MY SISTER MANAGED TO PULL THROUGH WITH NO HARD FEELINGS TOWARD ME—PROBABLY BECAUSE SHE WAS ONLY 4 YEARS OLD WHEN I GOT SICK, SO SHE DID NOT KNOW ANY BETTER. CHELLE WAS SENT TO EVERYONE'S HOUSE IN THE NEIGHBORHOOD SO THAT MY PARENTS WERE FREED UP TO CARE FOR ME. SHE DOESN'T REMEMBER MUCH OF IT NOW EXCEPT THAT I WASN'T AROUND OFTEN.
BYE, ALESIA! SEE YOU LATER, ALLIGATOR!

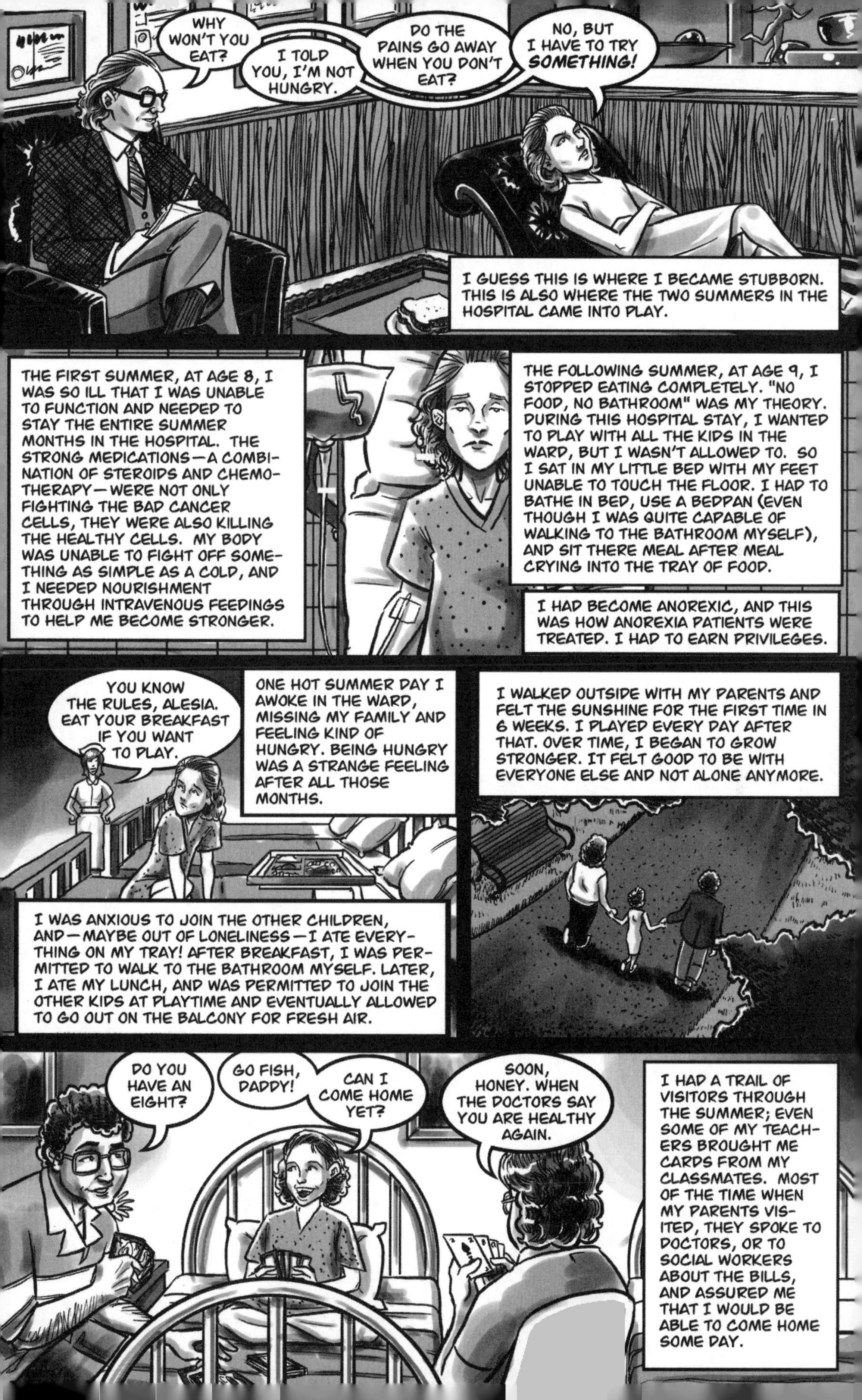
WHY WON'T YOU EAT?
I TOLD YOU, I'M NOT HUNGRY.
DO THE PAINS GO AWAY WHEN YOU DON'T EAT?
NO, BUT I HAVE TO TRY SOMETHING!
I GUESS THIS IS WHERE I BECAME STUBBORN. THIS IS ALSO WHERE THE TWO SUMMERS IN THE HOSPITAL CAME INTO PLAY.
THE FIRST SUMMER, AT AGE 8, I WAS SO ILL THAT I WAS UNABLE TO FUNCTION AND NEEDED TO STAY THE ENTIRE SUMMER MONTHS IN THE HOSPITAL. THE STRONG MEDICATIONS—A COMBINATION OF STEROIDS AND CHEMOTHERAPY—WERE NOT ONLY FIGHTING THE BAD CANCER CELLS, THEY WERE ALSO KILLING THE HEALTHY CELLS. MY BODY WAS UNABLE TO FIGHT OFF SOMETHING AS SIMPLE AS A COLD, AND I NEEDED NOURISHMENT THROUGH INTRAVENOUS FEEDINGS TO HELP ME BECOME STRONGER.
THE FOLLOWING SUMMER, AT AGE 9, I STOPPED EATING COMPLETELY. "NO FOOD, NO BATHROOM" WAS MY THEORY. DURING THIS HOSPITAL STAY, I WANTED TO PLAY WITH ALL THE KIDS IN THE WARD, BUT I WASN'T ALLOWED TO. SO I SAT IN MY LITTLE BED WITH MY FEET UNABLE TO TOUCH THE FLOOR. I HAD TO BATHE IN BED, USE A BEDPAN (EVEN THOUGH I WAS QUITE CAPABLE OF WALKING TO THE BATHROOM MYSELF), AND SIT THERE MEAL AFTER MEAL CRYING INTO THE TRAY OF FOOD.
I HAD BECOME ANOREXIC, AND THIS WAS HOW ANOREXIA PATIENTS WERE TREATED. I HAD TO EARN PRIVILEGES.
YOU KNOW THE RULES, ALESIA. EAT YOUR BREAKFAST IF YOU WANT TO PLAY.
ONE HOT SUMMER DAY I AWOKE IN THE WARD, MISSING MY FAMILY AND FEELING KIND OF HUNGRY. BEING HUNGRY WAS A STRANGE FEELING AFTER ALL THOSE MONTHS.
I WAS ANXIOUS TO JOIN THE OTHER CHILDREN, AND—MAYBE OUT OF LONELINESS—I ATE EVERYTHING ON MY TRAY! AFTER BREAKFAST, I WAS PERMITTED TO WALK TO THE BATHROOM MYSELF. LATER, I ATE MY LUNCH, AND WAS PERMITTED TO JOIN THE OTHER KIDS AT PLAYTIME AND EVENTUALLY ALLOWED TO GO OUT ON THE BALCONY FOR FRESH AIR.
I WALKED OUTSIDE WITH MY PARENTS AND FELT THE SUNSHINE FOR THE FIRST TIME IN 6 WEEKS. I PLAYED EVERY DAY AFTER THAT. OVER TIME, I BEGAN TO GROW STRONGER. IT FELT GOOD TO BE WITH EVERYONE ELSE AND NOT ALONE ANYMORE.
DO YOU HAVE AN EIGHT?
GO FISH, DADDY!
CAN I COME HOME YET?
SOON, HONEY. WHEN THE DOCTORS SAY YOU ARE HEALTHY AGAIN.
I HAD A TRAIL OF VISITORS THROUGH THE SUMMER; EVEN SOME OF MY TEACHERS BROUGHT ME CARDS FROM MY CLASSMATES. MOST OF THE TIME WHEN MY PARENTS VISITED, THEY SPOKE TO DOCTORS, OR TO SOCIAL WORKERS ABOUT THE BILLS, AND ASSURED ME THAT I WOULD BE ABLE TO COME HOME SOME DAY.

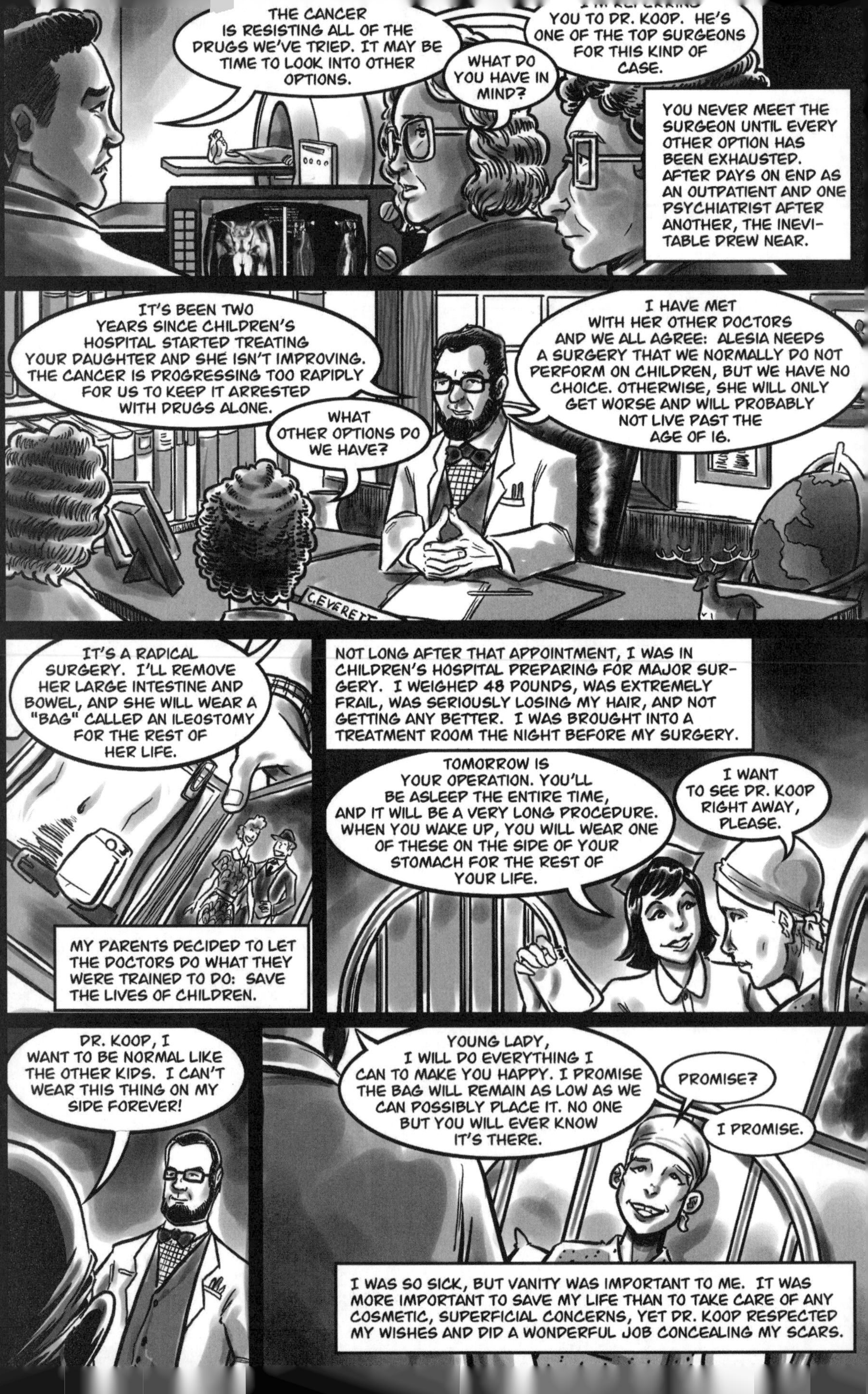
THE CANCER IS RESISTING ALL OF THE DRUGS WE'VE TRIED. IT MAY BE TIME TO LOOK INTO OTHER OPTIONS.
WHAT DO YOU HAVE IN MIND?
YOU TO DR. KOOP. HE'S ONE OF THE TOP SURGEONS FOR THIS KIND OF CASE.
YOU NEVER MEET THE SURGEON UNTIL EVERY OTHER OPTION HAS BEEN EXHAUSTED. AFTER DAYS ON END AS AN OUTPATIENT AND ONE PSYCHIATRIST AFTER ANOTHER, THE INEVITABLE DREW NEAR.
IT'S BEEN TWO YEARS SINCE CHILDREN'S HOSPITAL STARTED TREATING YOUR DAUGHTER AND SHE ISN'T IMPROVING. THE CANCER IS PROGRESSING TOO RAPIDLY FOR US TO KEEP IT ARRESTED WITH DRUGS ALONE.
WHAT OTHER OPTIONS DO WE HAVE?
I HAVE MET WITH HER OTHER DOCTORS AND WE ALL AGREE: ALESIA NEEDS A SURGERY THAT WE NORMALLY DO NOT PERFORM ON CHILDREN, BUT WE HAVE NO CHOICE. OTHERWISE, SHE WILL ONLY GET WORSE AND WILL PROBABLY NOT LIVE PAST THE AGE OF 16.
C.EVERETT
IT'S A RADICAL SURGERY. I'LL REMOVE HER LARGE INTESTINE AND BOWEL, AND SHE WILL WEAR A "BAG" CALLED AN ILEOSTOMY FOR THE REST OF HER LIFE.
MY PARENTS DECIDED TO LET THE DOCTORS DO WHAT THEY WERE TRAINED TO DO: SAVE THE LIVES OF CHILDREN.
NOT LONG AFTER THAT APPOINTMENT, I WAS IN CHILDREN'S HOSPITAL PREPARING FOR MAJOR SURGERY. I WEIGHED 48 POUNDS, WAS EXTREMELY FRAIL, WAS SERIOUSLY LOSING MY HAIR, AND NOT GETTING ANY BETTER. I WAS BROUGHT INTO A TREATMENT ROOM THE NIGHT BEFORE MY SURGERY.
TOMORROW IS YOUR OPERATION. YOU'LL BE ASLEEP THE ENTIRE TIME, AND IT WILL BE A VERY LONG PROCEDURE. WHEN YOU WAKE UP, YOU WILL WEAR ONE OF THESE ON THE SIDE OF YOUR STOMACH FOR THE REST OF YOUR LIFE.
I WANT TO SEE DR. KOOP RIGHT AWAY, PLEASE.
DR. KOOP, I WANT TO BE NORMAL LIKE THE OTHER KIDS. I CAN'T WEAR THIS THING ON MY SIDE FOREVER!
YOUNG LADY, I WILL DO EVERYTHING I CAN TO MAKE YOU HAPPY. I PROMISE THE BAG WILL REMAIN AS LOW AS WE CAN POSSIBLY PLACE IT. NO ONE BUT YOU WILL EVER KNOW IT'S THERE.
PROMISE?
I PROMISE.
I WAS SO SICK, BUT VANITY WAS IMPORTANT TO ME. IT WAS MORE IMPORTANT TO SAVE MY LIFE THAN TO TAKE CARE OF ANY COSMETIC, SUPERFICIAL CONCERNS, YET DR. KOOP RESPECTED MY WISHES AND DID A WONDERFUL JOB CONCEALING MY SCARS.

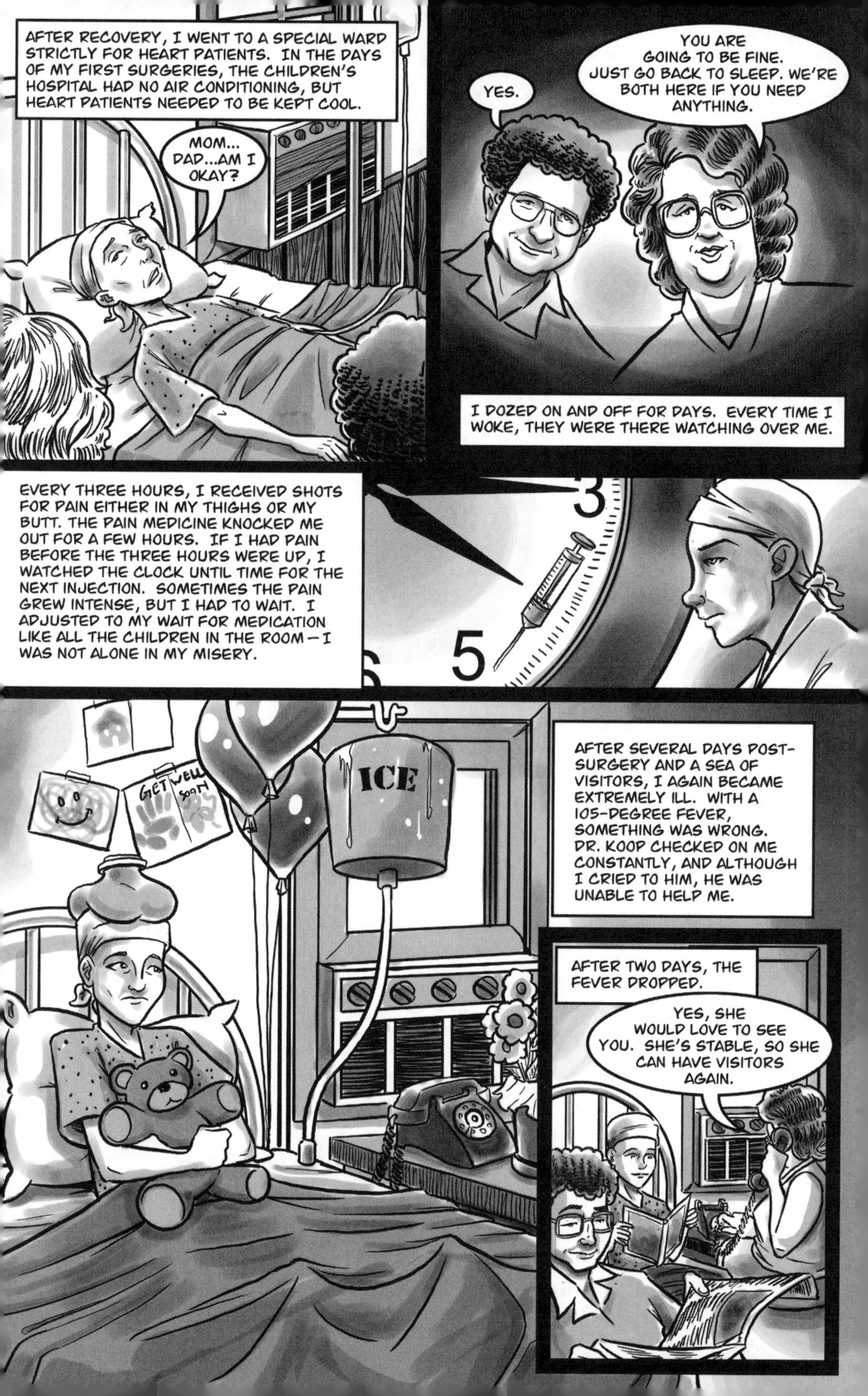
AFTER RECOVERY, I WENT TO A SPECIAL WARD STRICTLY FOR HEART PATIENTS. IN THE DAYS OF MY FIRST SURGERIES, THE CHILDREN'S HOSPITAL HAD NO AIR CONDITIONING, BUT HEART PATIENTS NEEDED TO BE KEPT COOL.
MOM... DAD...AM I OKAY?
YES.
YOU ARE GOING TO BE FINE. JUST GO BACK TO SLEEP. WE'RE BOTH HERE IF YOU NEED ANYTHING.
I DOZED ON AND OFF FOR DAYS. EVERY TIME I WOKE, THEY WERE THERE WATCHING OVER ME.
EVERY THREE HOURS, I RECEIVED SHOTS FOR PAIN EITHER IN MY THIGHS OR MY BUTT. THE PAIN MEDICINE KNOCKED ME OUT FOR A FEW HOURS. IF I HAD PAIN BEFORE THE THREE HOURS WERE UP, I WATCHED THE CLOCK UNTIL TIME FOR THE NEXT INJECTION. SOMETIMES THE PAIN GREW INTENSE, BUT I HAD TO WAIT. I ADJUSTED TO MY WAIT FOR MEDICATION LIKE ALL THE CHILDREN IN THE ROOM — I WAS NOT ALONE IN MY MISERY.
3
5
GET WELL Soon
ICE
AFTER SEVERAL DAYS POST-SURGERY AND A SEA OF VISITORS, I AGAIN BECAME EXTREMELY ILL. WITH A 105-DEGREE FEVER, SOMETHING WAS WRONG. DR. KOOP CHECKED ON ME CONSTANTLY, AND ALTHOUGH I CRIED TO HIM, HE WAS UNABLE TO HELP ME.
AFTER TWO DAYS, THE FEVER DROPPED.
YES, SHE WOULD LOVE TO SEE YOU. SHE'S STABLE, SO SHE CAN HAVE VISITORS AGAIN.

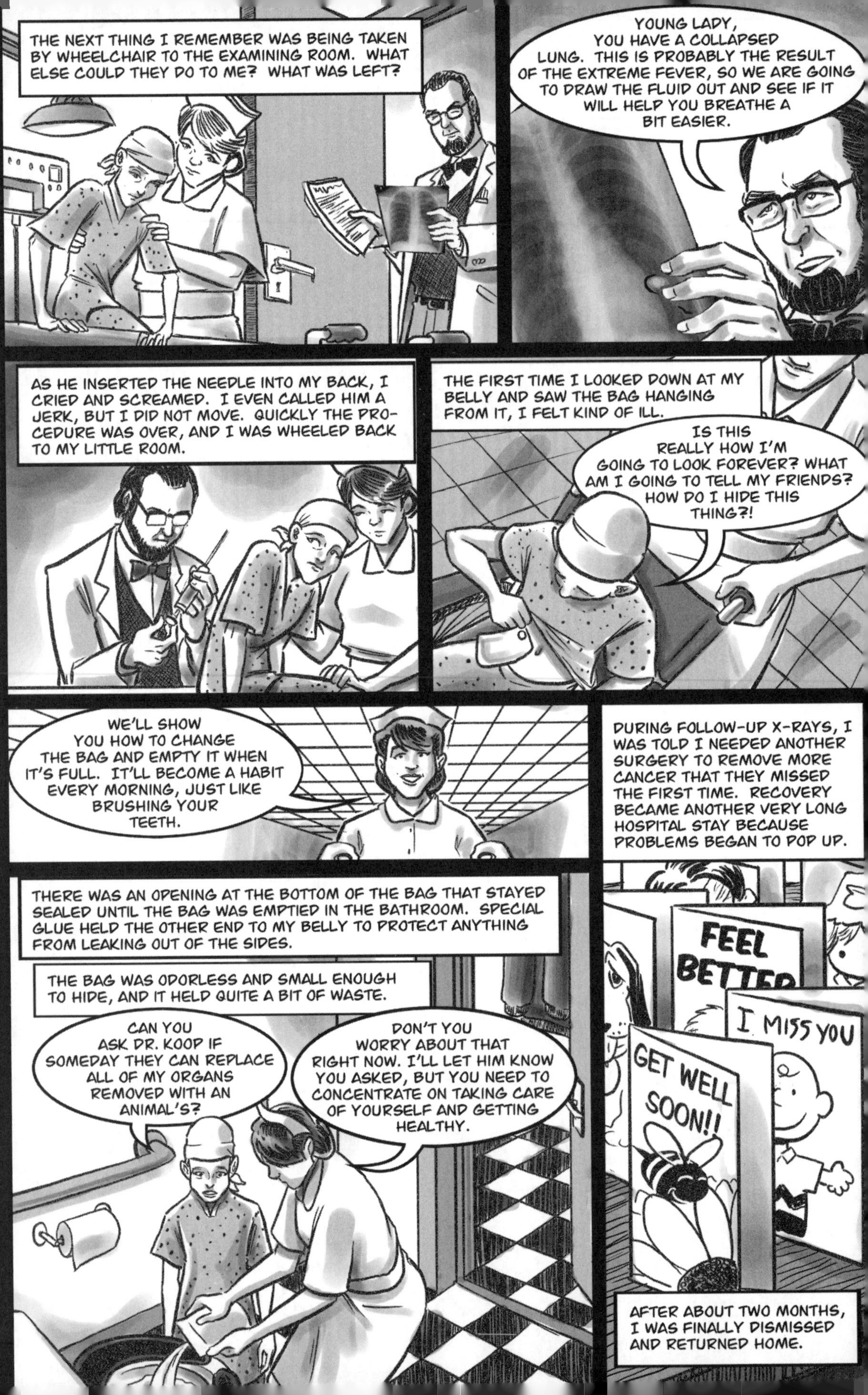
THE NEXT THING I REMEMBER WAS BEING TAKEN BY WHEELCHAIR TO THE EXAMINING ROOM. WHAT ELSE COULD THEY DO TO ME? WHAT WAS LEFT?
YOUNG LADY, YOU HAVE A COLLAPSED LUNG. THIS IS PROBABLY THE RESULT OF THE EXTREME FEVER, SO WE ARE GOING TO DRAW THE FLUID OUT AND SEE IF IT WILL HELP YOU BREATHE A BIT EASIER.
AS HE INSERTED THE NEEDLE INTO MY BACK, I CRIED AND SCREAMED. I EVEN CALLED HIM A JERK, BUT I DID NOT MOVE. QUICKLY THE PROCEDURE WAS OVER, AND I WAS WHEELED BACK TO MY LITTLE ROOM.
THE FIRST TIME I LOOKED DOWN AT MY BELLY AND SAW THE BAG HANGING FROM IT, I FELT KIND OF ILL.
IS THIS REALLY HOW I'M GOING TO LOOK FOREVER? WHAT AM I GOING TO TELL MY FRIENDS? HOW DO I HIDE THIS THING?!
WE'LL SHOW YOU HOW TO CHANGE THE BAG AND EMPTY IT WHEN IT'S FULL. IT'LL BECOME A HABIT EVERY MORNING, JUST LIKE BRUSHING YOUR TEETH.
DURING FOLLOW-UP X-RAYS, I WAS TOLD I NEEDED ANOTHER SURGERY TO REMOVE MORE CANCER THAT THEY MISSED THE FIRST TIME. RECOVERY BECAME ANOTHER VERY LONG HOSPITAL STAY BECAUSE PROBLEMS BEGAN TO POP UP.
THERE WAS AN OPENING AT THE BOTTOM OF THE BAG THAT STAYED SEALED UNTIL THE BAG WAS EMPTIED IN THE BATHROOM. SPECIAL GLUE HELD THE OTHER END TO MY BELLY TO PROTECT ANYTHING FROM LEAKING OUT OF THE SIDES.
THE BAG WAS ODORLESS AND SMALL ENOUGH TO HIDE, AND IT HELD QUITE A BIT OF WASTE.
CAN YOU ASK DR. KOOP IF SOMEDAY THEY CAN REPLACE ALL OF MY ORGANS REMOVED WITH AN ANIMAL'S?
DON'T YOU WORRY ABOUT THAT RIGHT NOW. I'LL LET HIM KNOW YOU ASKED, BUT YOU NEED TO CONCENTRATE ON TAKING CARE OF YOURSELF AND GETTING HEALTHY.
FEEL BETTER
I MISS YOU
GET WELL SOON!!
AFTER ABOUT TWO MONTHS, I WAS FINALLY DISMISSED AND RETURNED HOME.

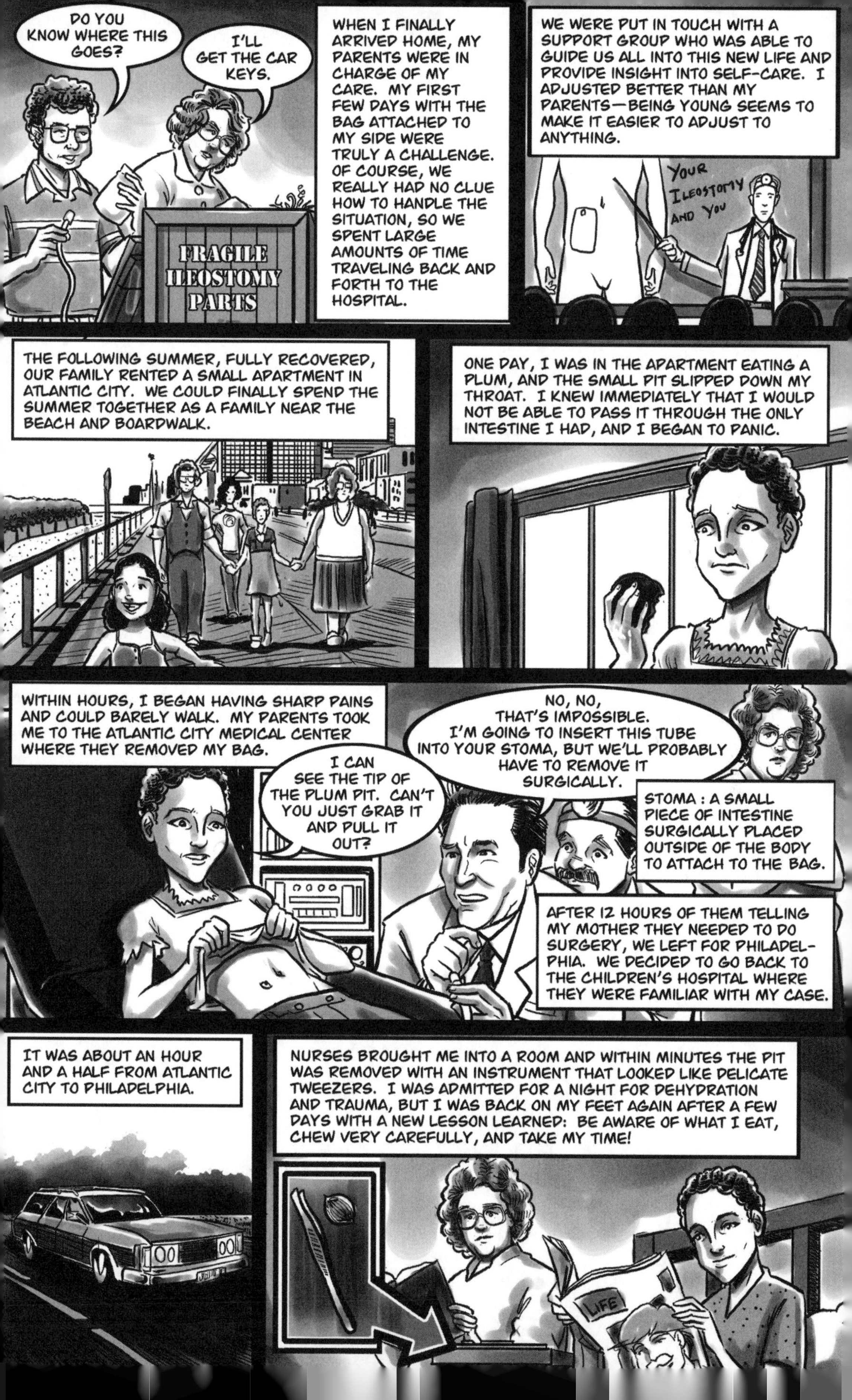
DO YOU KNOW WHERE THIS GOES?
I'LL GET THE CAR KEYS.
FRAGILE ILEOSTOMY PARTS
WHEN I FINALLY ARRIVED HOME, MY PARENTS WERE IN CHARGE OF MY CARE. MY FIRST FEW DAYS WITH THE BAG ATTACHED TO MY SIDE WERE TRULY A CHALLENGE. OF COURSE, WE REALLY HAD NO CLUE HOW TO HANDLE THE SITUATION, SO WE SPENT LARGE AMOUNTS OF TIME TRAVELING BACK AND FORTH TO THE HOSPITAL.
WE WERE PUT IN TOUCH WITH A SUPPORT GROUP WHO WAS ABLE TO GUIDE US ALL INTO THIS NEW LIFE AND PROVIDE INSIGHT INTO SELF-CARE. I ADJUSTED BETTER THAN MY PARENTS—BEING YOUNG SEEMS TO MAKE IT EASIER TO ADJUST TO ANYTHING.
YOUR ILEOSTOMY AND YOU
THE FOLLOWING SUMMER, FULLY RECOVERED, OUR FAMILY RENTED A SMALL APARTMENT IN ATLANTIC CITY. WE COULD FINALLY SPEND THE SUMMER TOGETHER AS A FAMILY NEAR THE BEACH AND BOARDWALK.
ONE DAY, I WAS IN THE APARTMENT EATING A PLUM, AND THE SMALL PIT SLIPPED DOWN MY THROAT. I KNEW IMMEDIATELY THAT I WOULD NOT BE ABLE TO PASS IT THROUGH THE ONLY INTESTINE I HAD, AND I BEGAN TO PANIC.
WITHIN HOURS, I BEGAN HAVING SHARP PAINS AND COULD BARELY WALK. MY PARENTS TOOK ME TO THE ATLANTIC CITY MEDICAL CENTER WHERE THEY REMOVED MY BAG.
I CAN SEE THE TIP OF THE PLUM PIT. CAN'T YOU JUST GRAB IT AND PULL IT OUT?
NO, NO, THAT'S IMPOSSIBLE. I'M GOING TO INSERT THIS TUBE INTO YOUR STOMA, BUT WE'LL PROBABLY HAVE TO REMOVE IT SURGICALLY.
STOMA : A SMALL PIECE OF INTESTINE SURGICALLY PLACED OUTSIDE OF THE BODY TO ATTACH TO THE BAG.
AFTER 12 HOURS OF THEM TELLING MY MOTHER THEY NEEDED TO DO SURGERY, WE LEFT FOR PHILADEL-PHIA. WE DECIDED TO GO BACK TO THE CHILDREN'S HOSPITAL WHERE THEY WERE FAMILIAR WITH MY CASE.
IT WAS ABOUT AN HOUR AND A HALF FROM ATLANTIC CITY TO PHILADELPHIA.
NURSES BROUGHT ME INTO A ROOM AND WITHIN MINUTES THE PIT WAS REMOVED WITH AN INSTRUMENT THAT LOOKED LIKE DELICATE TWEEZERS. I WAS ADMITTED FOR A NIGHT FOR DEHYDRATION AND TRAUMA, BUT I WAS BACK ON MY FEET AGAIN AFTER A FEW DAYS WITH A NEW LESSON LEARNED: BE AWARE OF WHAT I EAT, CHEW VERY CAREFULLY, AND TAKE MY TIME!
LIFE

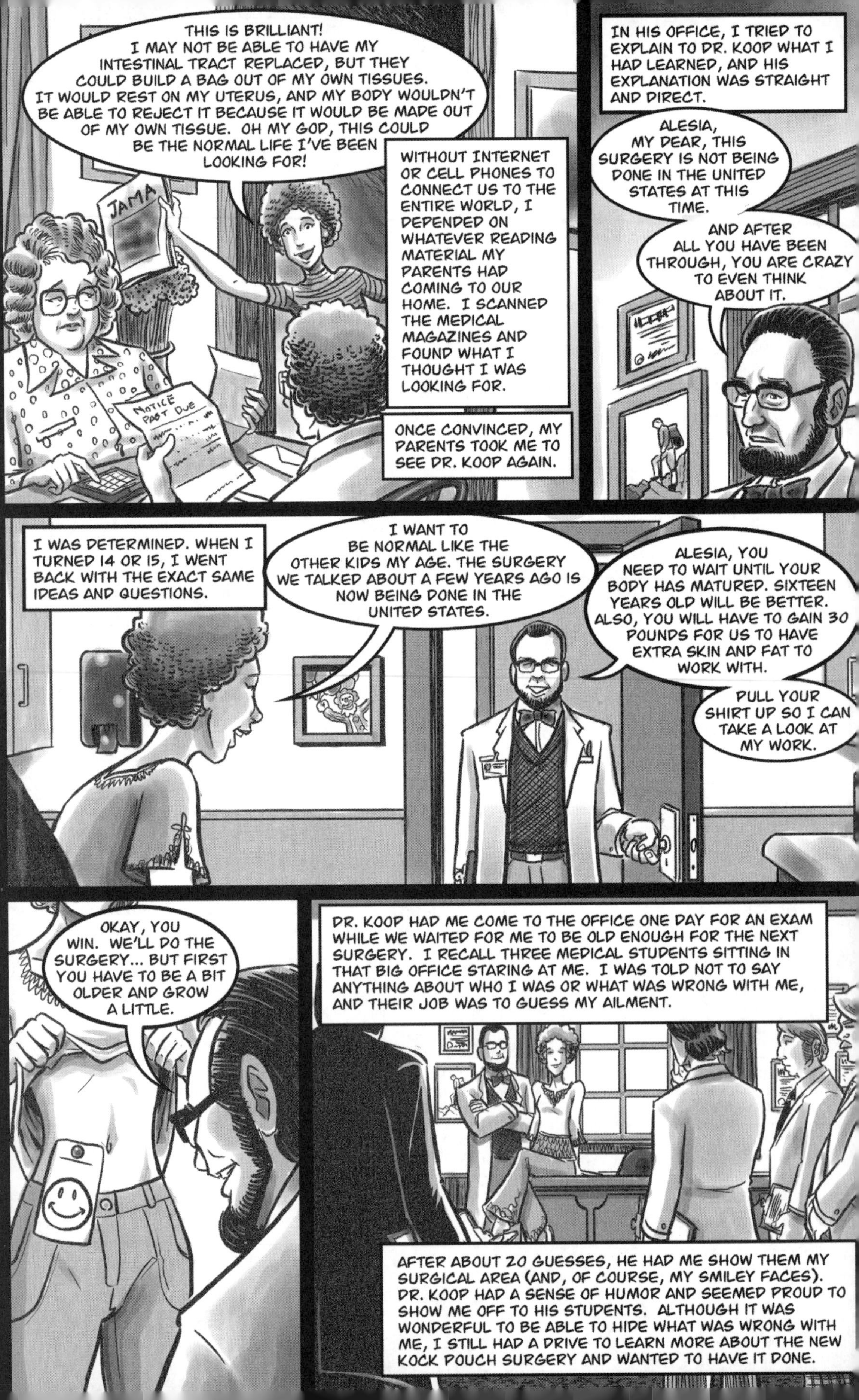
THIS IS BRILLIANT! I MAY NOT BE ABLE TO HAVE MY INTESTINAL TRACT REPLACED, BUT THEY COULD BUILD A BAG OUT OF MY OWN TISSUES. IT WOULD REST ON MY UTERUS, AND MY BODY WOULDN'T BE ABLE TO REJECT IT BECAUSE IT WOULD BE MADE OUT OF MY OWN TISSUE. OH MY GOD, THIS COULD BE THE NORMAL LIFE I'VE BEEN LOOKING FOR!
JAMA
NOTICE PAST DUE
WITHOUT INTERNET OR CELL PHONES TO CONNECT US TO THE ENTIRE WORLD, I DEPENDED ON WHATEVER READING MATERIAL MY PARENTS HAD COMING TO OUR HOME. I SCANNED THE MEDICAL MAGAZINES AND FOUND WHAT I THOUGHT I WAS LOOKING FOR.
ONCE CONVINCED, MY PARENTS TOOK ME TO SEE DR. KOOP AGAIN.
IN HIS OFFICE, I TRIED TO EXPLAIN TO DR. KOOP WHAT I HAD LEARNED, AND HIS EXPLANATION WAS STRAIGHT AND DIRECT.
ALESIA, MY DEAR, THIS SURGERY IS NOT BEING DONE IN THE UNITED STATES AT THIS TIME.
AND AFTER ALL YOU HAVE BEEN THROUGH, YOU ARE CRAZY TO EVEN THINK ABOUT IT.
I WAS DETERMINED. WHEN I TURNED 14 OR 15, I WENT BACK WITH THE EXACT SAME IDEAS AND QUESTIONS.
I WANT TO BE NORMAL LIKE THE OTHER KIDS MY AGE. THE SURGERY WE TALKED ABOUT A FEW YEARS AGO IS NOW BEING DONE IN THE UNITED STATES.
ALESIA, YOU NEED TO WAIT UNTIL YOUR BODY HAS MATURED. SIXTEEN YEARS OLD WILL BE BETTER. ALSO, YOU WILL HAVE TO GAIN 30 POUNDS FOR US TO HAVE EXTRA SKIN AND FAT TO WORK WITH.
PULL YOUR SHIRT UP SO I CAN TAKE A LOOK AT MY WORK.
OKAY, YOU WIN. WE'LL DO THE SURGERY... BUT FIRST YOU HAVE TO BE A BIT OLDER AND GROW A LITTLE.
DR. KOOP HAD ME COME TO THE OFFICE ONE DAY FOR AN EXAM WHILE WE WAITED FOR ME TO BE OLD ENOUGH FOR THE NEXT SURGERY. I RECALL THREE MEDICAL STUDENTS SITTING IN THAT BIG OFFICE STARING AT ME. I WAS TOLD NOT TO SAY ANYTHING ABOUT WHO I WAS OR WHAT WAS WRONG WITH ME, AND THEIR JOB WAS TO GUESS MY AILMENT.
AFTER ABOUT 20 GUESSES, HE HAD ME SHOW THEM MY SURGICAL AREA (AND, OF COURSE, MY SMILEY FACES). DR. KOOP HAD A SENSE OF HUMOR AND SEEMED PROUD TO SHOW ME OFF TO HIS STUDENTS. ALTHOUGH IT WAS WONDERFUL TO BE ABLE TO HIDE WHAT WAS WRONG WITH ME, I STILL HAD A DRIVE TO LEARN MORE ABOUT THE NEW KOCK POUCH SURGERY AND WANTED TO HAVE IT DONE.

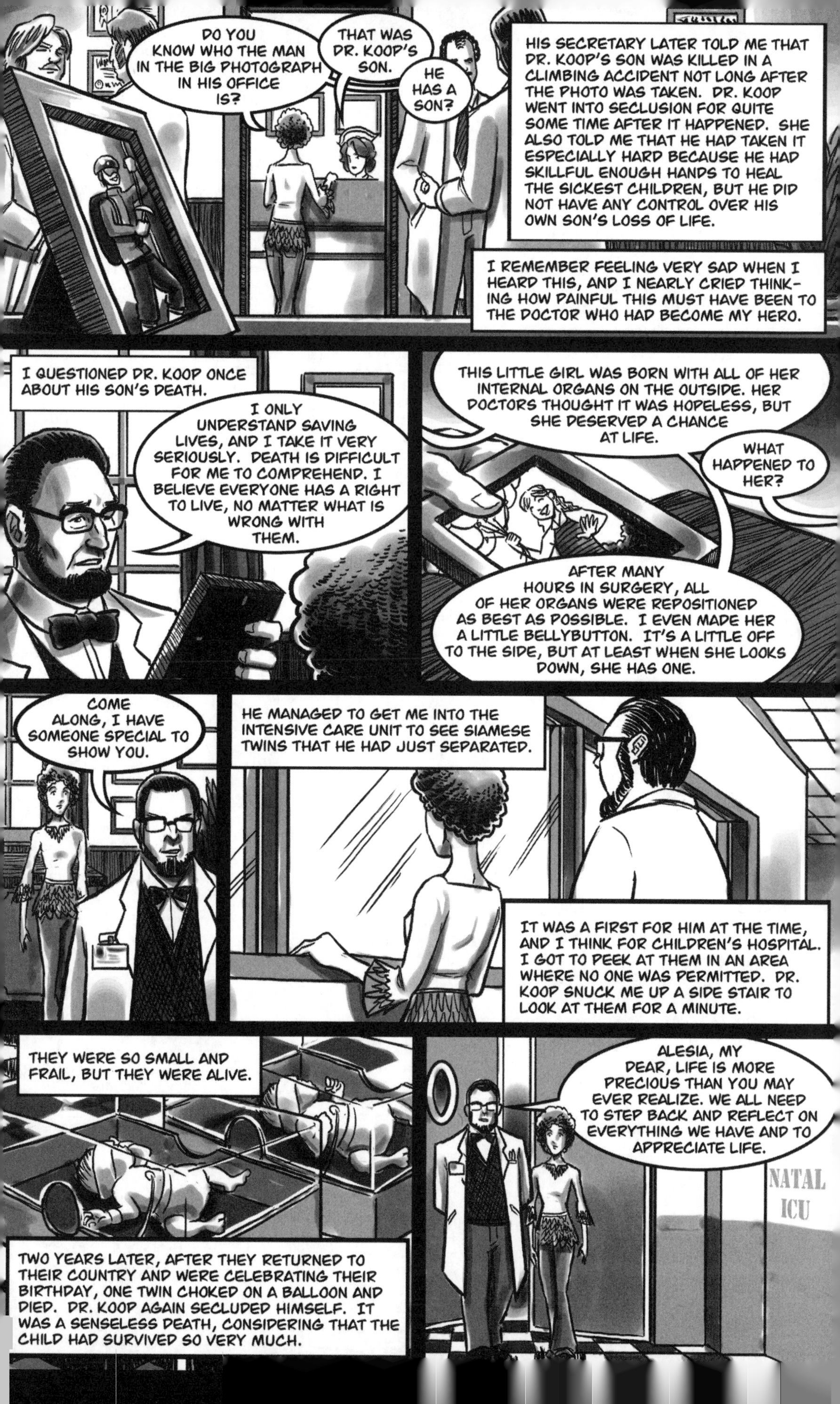

DO YOU KNOW WHO THE MAN IN THE BIG PHOTOGRAPH IN HIS OFFICE IS?
THAT WAS DR. KOOP'S SON.
HE HAS A SON?
HIS SECRETARY LATER TOLD ME THAT DR. KOOP'S SON WAS KILLED IN A CLIMBING ACCIDENT NOT LONG AFTER THE PHOTO WAS TAKEN. DR. KOOP WENT INTO SECLUSION FOR QUITE SOME TIME AFTER IT HAPPENED. SHE ALSO TOLD ME THAT HE HAD TAKEN IT ESPECIALLY HARD BECAUSE HE HAD SKILLFUL ENOUGH HANDS TO HEAL THE SICKEST CHILDREN, BUT HE DID NOT HAVE ANY CONTROL OVER HIS OWN SON'S LOSS OF LIFE.
I REMEMBER FEELING VERY SAD WHEN I HEARD THIS, AND I NEARLY CRIED THINKING HOW PAINFUL THIS MUST HAVE BEEN TO THE DOCTOR WHO HAD BECOME MY HERO.
I QUESTIONED DR. KOOP ONCE ABOUT HIS SON'S DEATH.
I ONLY UNDERSTAND SAVING LIVES, AND I TAKE IT VERY SERIOUSLY. DEATH IS DIFFICULT FOR ME TO COMPREHEND. I BELIEVE EVERYONE HAS A RIGHT TO LIVE, NO MATTER WHAT IS WRONG WITH THEM.
THIS LITTLE GIRL WAS BORN WITH ALL OF HER INTERNAL ORGANS ON THE OUTSIDE. HER DOCTORS THOUGHT IT WAS HOPELESS, BUT SHE DESERVED A CHANCE AT LIFE.
WHAT HAPPENED TO HER?
AFTER MANY HOURS IN SURGERY, ALL OF HER ORGANS WERE REPOSITIONED AS BEST AS POSSIBLE. I EVEN MADE HER A LITTLE BELLYBUTTON. IT'S A LITTLE OFF TO THE SIDE, BUT AT LEAST WHEN SHE LOOKS DOWN, SHE HAS ONE.
COME ALONG, I HAVE SOMEONE SPECIAL TO SHOW YOU.
HE MANAGED TO GET ME INTO THE INTENSIVE CARE UNIT TO SEE SIAMESE TWINS THAT HE HAD JUST SEPARATED.
IT WAS A FIRST FOR HIM AT THE TIME, AND I THINK FOR CHILDREN'S HOSPITAL. I GOT TO PEEK AT THEM IN AN AREA WHERE NO ONE WAS PERMITTED. DR. KOOP SNUCK ME UP A SIDE STAIR TO LOOK AT THEM FOR A MINUTE.
THEY WERE SO SMALL AND FRAIL, BUT THEY WERE ALIVE.
TWO YEARS LATER, AFTER THEY RETURNED TO THEIR COUNTRY AND WERE CELEBRATING THEIR BIRTHDAY, ONE TWIN CHOKED ON A BALLOON AND DIED. DR. KOOP AGAIN SECLUDED HIMSELF. IT WAS A SENSELESS DEATH, CONSIDERING THAT THE CHILD HAD SURVIVED SO VERY MUCH.
ALESIA, MY DEAR, LIFE IS MORE PRECIOUS THAN YOU MAY EVER REALIZE. WE ALL NEED TO STEP BACK AND REFLECT ON EVERYTHING WE HAVE AND TO APPRECIATE LIFE.
NATAL ICU

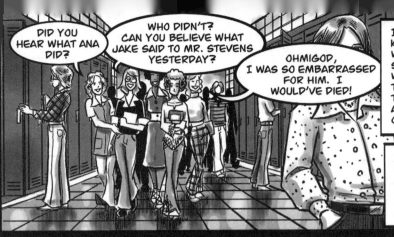

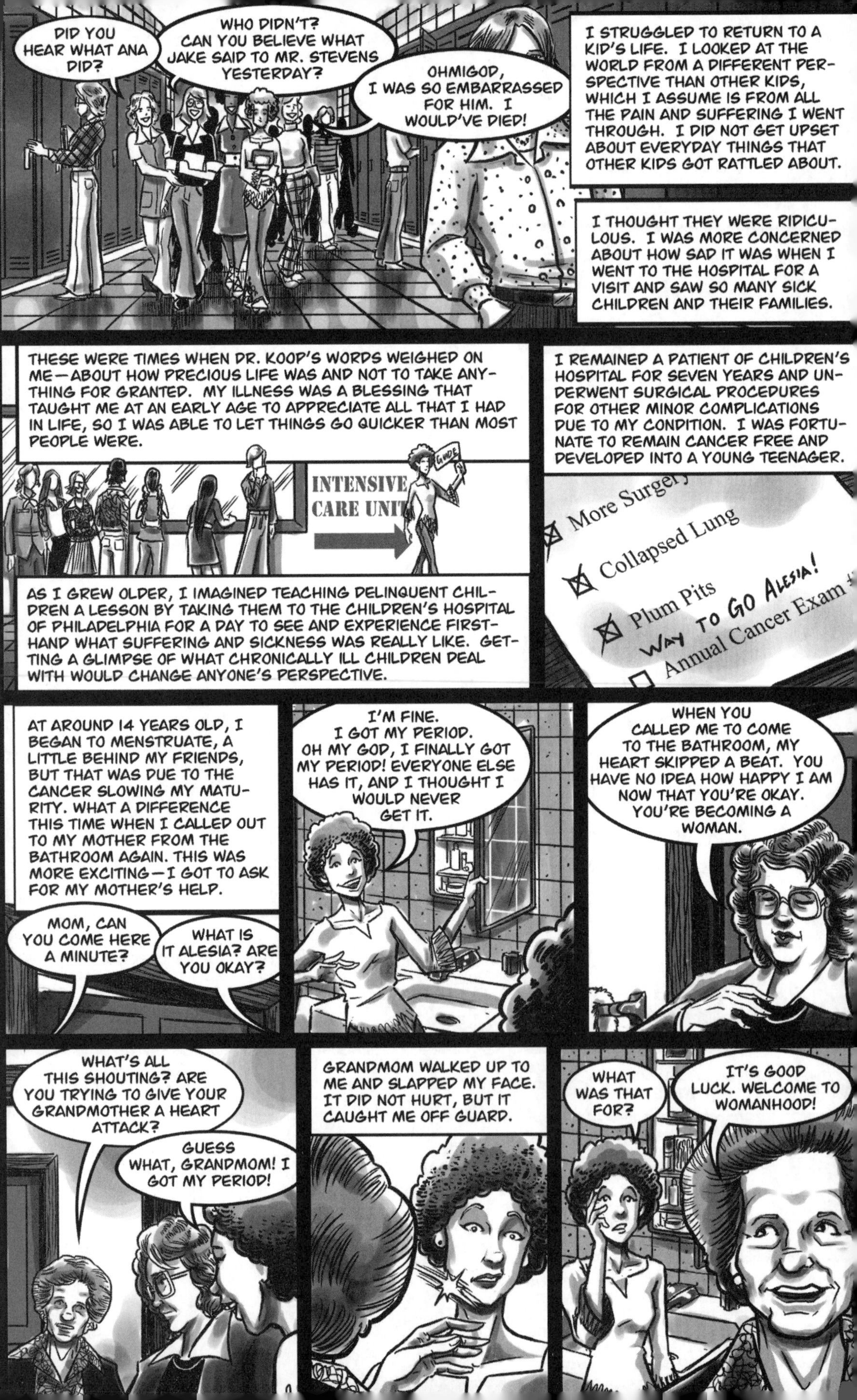

DID YOU HEAR WHAT ANA DID?

WHO DIDN'T? CAN YOU BELIEVE WHAT JAKE SAID TO MR. STEVENS YESTERDAY?

OHMIGOD, I WAS SO EMBARRASSED FOR HIM. I WOULD'VE DIED!

I STRUGGLED TO RETURN TO A KID'S LIFE. I LOOKED AT THE WORLD FROM A DIFFERENT PERSPECTIVE THAN OTHER KIDS, WHICH I ASSUME IS FROM ALL THE PAIN AND SUFFERING I WENT THROUGH. I DID NOT GET UPSET ABOUT EVERYDAY THINGS THAT OTHER KIDS GOT RATTLED ABOUT.

I THOUGHT THEY WERE RIDICULOUS. I WAS MORE CONCERNED ABOUT HOW SAD IT WAS WHEN I WENT TO THE HOSPITAL FOR A VISIT AND SAW SO MANY SICK CHILDREN AND THEIR FAMILIES.

THESE WERE TIMES WHEN DR. KOOP'S WORDS WEIGHED ON ME—ABOUT HOW PRECIOUS LIFE WAS AND NOT TO TAKE ANYTHING FOR GRANTED. MY ILLNESS WAS A BLESSING THAT TAUGHT ME AT AN EARLY AGE TO APPRECIATE ALL THAT I HAD IN LIFE, SO I WAS ABLE TO LET THINGS GO QUICKER THAN MOST PEOPLE WERE.

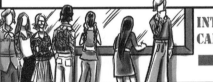

INTENSIVE CARE UNIT

I REMAINED A PATIENT OF CHILDREN'S HOSPITAL FOR SEVEN YEARS AND UNDERWENT SURGICAL PROCEDURES FOR OTHER MINOR COMPLICATIONS DUE TO MY CONDITION. I WAS FORTUNATE TO REMAIN CANCER FREE AND DEVELOPED INTO A YOUNG TEENAGER.

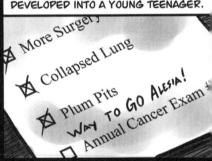

☒ More Surgery
☒ Collapsed Lung
☒ Plum Pits
WAY TO GO ALESIA!
☐ Annual Cancer Exam

AS I GREW OLDER, I IMAGINED TEACHING DELINQUENT CHILDREN A LESSON BY TAKING THEM TO THE CHILDREN'S HOSPITAL OF PHILADELPHIA FOR A DAY TO SEE AND EXPERIENCE FIRSTHAND WHAT SUFFERING AND SICKNESS WAS REALLY LIKE. GETTING A GLIMPSE OF WHAT CHRONICALLY ILL CHILDREN DEAL WITH WOULD CHANGE ANYONE'S PERSPECTIVE.

AT AROUND 14 YEARS OLD, I BEGAN TO MENSTRUATE, A LITTLE BEHIND MY FRIENDS, BUT THAT WAS DUE TO THE CANCER SLOWING MY MATURITY. WHAT A DIFFERENCE THIS TIME WHEN I CALLED OUT TO MY MOTHER FROM THE BATHROOM AGAIN. THIS WAS MORE EXCITING—I GOT TO ASK FOR MY MOTHER'S HELP.

MOM, CAN YOU COME HERE A MINUTE?

WHAT IS IT ALESIA? ARE YOU OKAY?

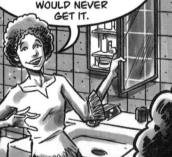

I'M FINE. I GOT MY PERIOD. OH MY GOD, I FINALLY GOT MY PERIOD! EVERYONE ELSE HAS IT, AND I THOUGHT I WOULD NEVER GET IT.

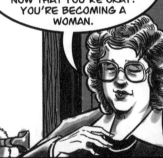

WHEN YOU CALLED ME TO COME TO THE BATHROOM, MY HEART SKIPPED A BEAT. YOU HAVE NO IDEA HOW HAPPY I AM NOW THAT YOU'RE OKAY. YOU'RE BECOMING A WOMAN.

WHAT'S ALL THIS SHOUTING? ARE YOU TRYING TO GIVE YOUR GRANDMOTHER A HEART ATTACK?

GUESS WHAT, GRANDMOM! I GOT MY PERIOD!

GRANDMOM WALKED UP TO ME AND SLAPPED MY FACE. IT DID NOT HURT, BUT IT CAUGHT ME OFF GUARD.

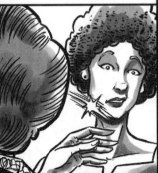

WHAT WAS THAT FOR?

IT'S GOOD LUCK. WELCOME TO WOMANHOOD!

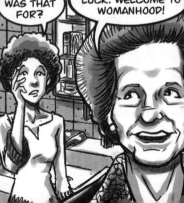

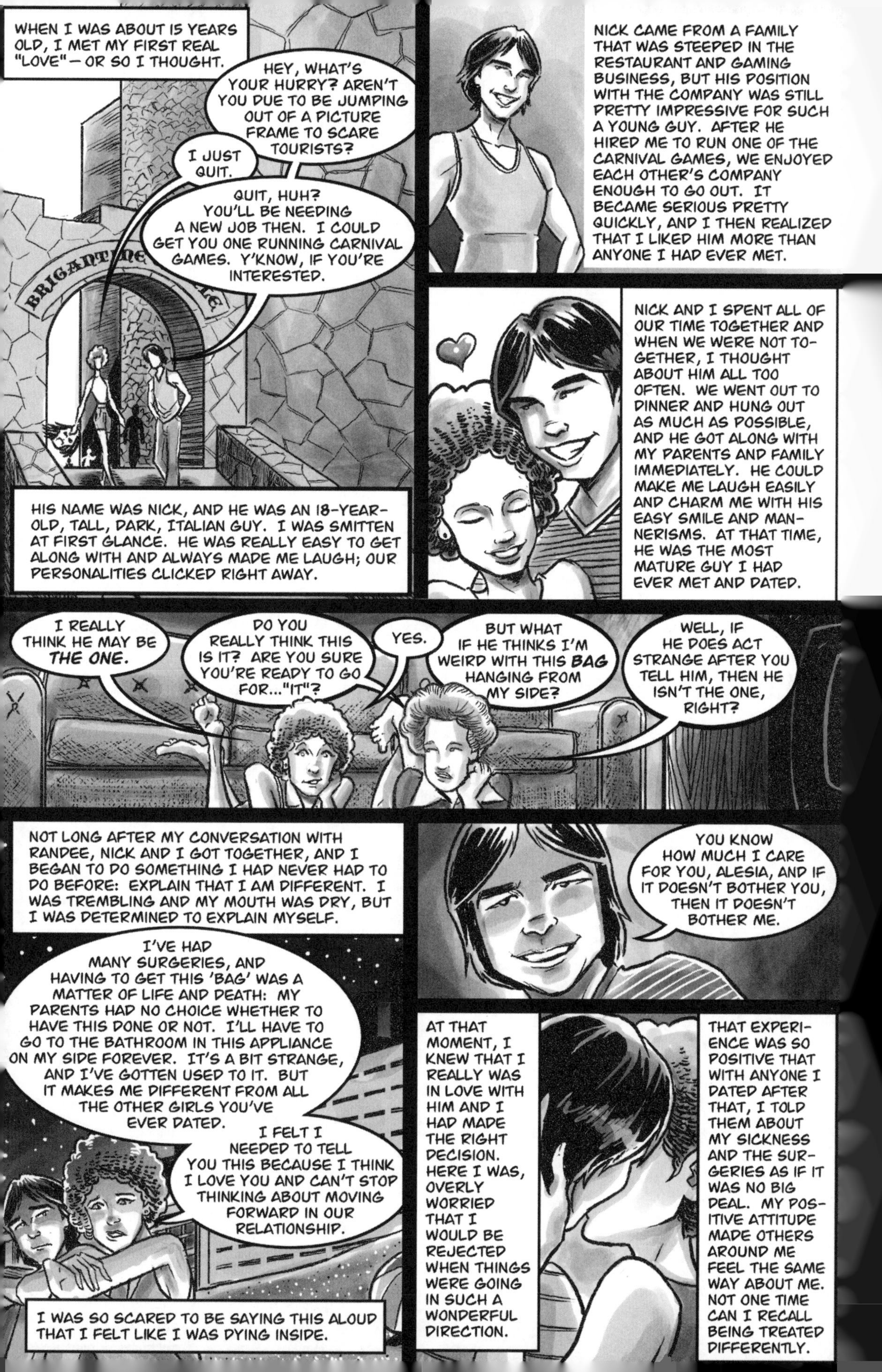
WHEN I WAS ABOUT 15 YEARS OLD, I MET MY FIRST REAL "LOVE"—OR SO I THOUGHT.
HEY, WHAT'S YOUR HURRY? AREN'T YOU DUE TO BE JUMPING OUT OF A PICTURE FRAME TO SCARE TOURISTS?
I JUST QUIT.
QUIT, HUH? YOU'LL BE NEEDING A NEW JOB THEN. I COULD GET YOU ONE RUNNING CARNIVAL GAMES. Y'KNOW, IF YOU'RE INTERESTED.
HIS NAME WAS NICK, AND HE WAS AN 18-YEAR-OLD, TALL, DARK, ITALIAN GUY. I WAS SMITTEN AT FIRST GLANCE. HE WAS REALLY EASY TO GET ALONG WITH AND ALWAYS MADE ME LAUGH; OUR PERSONALITIES CLICKED RIGHT AWAY.
NICK CAME FROM A FAMILY THAT WAS STEEPED IN THE RESTAURANT AND GAMING BUSINESS, BUT HIS POSITION WITH THE COMPANY WAS STILL PRETTY IMPRESSIVE FOR SUCH A YOUNG GUY. AFTER HE HIRED ME TO RUN ONE OF THE CARNIVAL GAMES, WE ENJOYED EACH OTHER'S COMPANY ENOUGH TO GO OUT. IT BECAME SERIOUS PRETTY QUICKLY, AND I THEN REALIZED THAT I LIKED HIM MORE THAN ANYONE I HAD EVER MET.
NICK AND I SPENT ALL OF OUR TIME TOGETHER AND WHEN WE WERE NOT TOGETHER, I THOUGHT ABOUT HIM ALL TOO OFTEN. WE WENT OUT TO DINNER AND HUNG OUT AS MUCH AS POSSIBLE, AND HE GOT ALONG WITH MY PARENTS AND FAMILY IMMEDIATELY. HE COULD MAKE ME LAUGH EASILY AND CHARM ME WITH HIS EASY SMILE AND MANNERISMS. AT THAT TIME, HE WAS THE MOST MATURE GUY I HAD EVER MET AND DATED.
I REALLY THINK HE MAY BE ***THE ONE.***
DO YOU REALLY THINK THIS IS IT? ARE YOU SURE YOU'RE READY TO GO FOR..."IT"?
YES.
BUT WHAT IF HE THINKS I'M WEIRD WITH THIS **BAG** HANGING FROM MY SIDE?
WELL, IF HE DOES ACT STRANGE AFTER YOU TELL HIM, THEN HE ISN'T THE ONE, RIGHT?
NOT LONG AFTER MY CONVERSATION WITH RANDEE, NICK AND I GOT TOGETHER, AND I BEGAN TO DO SOMETHING I HAD NEVER HAD TO DO BEFORE: EXPLAIN THAT I AM DIFFERENT. I WAS TREMBLING AND MY MOUTH WAS DRY, BUT I WAS DETERMINED TO EXPLAIN MYSELF.
I'VE HAD MANY SURGERIES, AND HAVING TO GET THIS 'BAG' WAS A MATTER OF LIFE AND DEATH: MY PARENTS HAD NO CHOICE WHETHER TO HAVE THIS DONE OR NOT. I'LL HAVE TO GO TO THE BATHROOM IN THIS APPLIANCE ON MY SIDE FOREVER. IT'S A BIT STRANGE, AND I'VE GOTTEN USED TO IT. BUT IT MAKES ME DIFFERENT FROM ALL THE OTHER GIRLS YOU'VE EVER DATED.
I FELT I NEEDED TO TELL YOU THIS BECAUSE I THINK I LOVE YOU AND CAN'T STOP THINKING ABOUT MOVING FORWARD IN OUR RELATIONSHIP.
I WAS SO SCARED TO BE SAYING THIS ALOUD THAT I FELT LIKE I WAS DYING INSIDE.
YOU KNOW HOW MUCH I CARE FOR YOU, ALESIA, AND IF IT DOESN'T BOTHER YOU, THEN IT DOESN'T BOTHER ME.
AT THAT MOMENT, I KNEW THAT I REALLY WAS IN LOVE WITH HIM AND I HAD MADE THE RIGHT DECISION. HERE I WAS, OVERLY WORRIED THAT I WOULD BE REJECTED WHEN THINGS WERE GOING IN SUCH A WONDERFUL DIRECTION.
THAT EXPERIENCE WAS SO POSITIVE THAT WITH ANYONE I DATED AFTER THAT, I TOLD THEM ABOUT MY SICKNESS AND THE SURGERIES AS IF IT WAS NO BIG DEAL. MY POSITIVE ATTITUDE MADE OTHERS AROUND ME FEEL THE SAME WAY ABOUT ME. NOT ONE TIME CAN I RECALL BEING TREATED DIFFERENTLY.

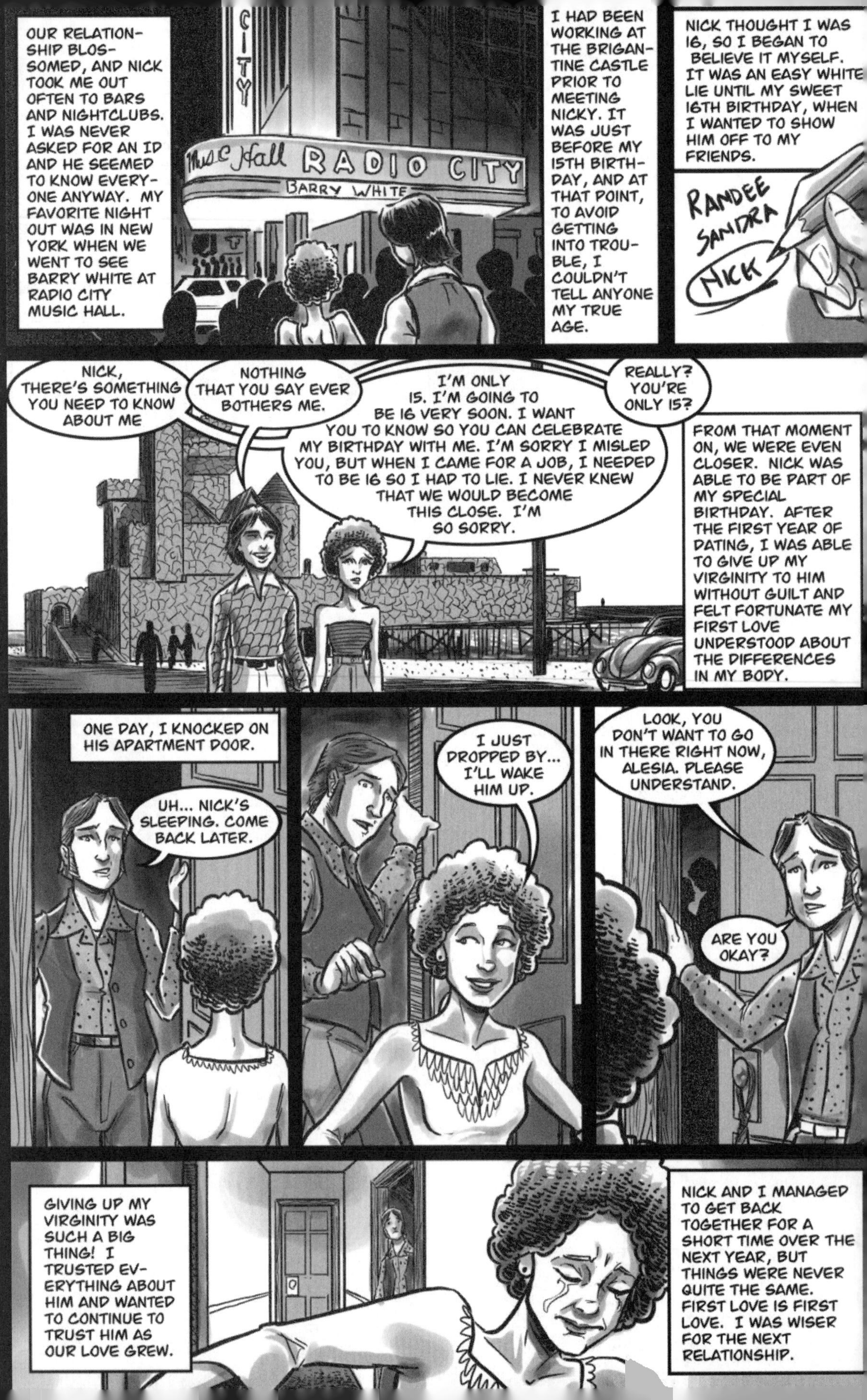
OUR RELATIONSHIP BLOSSOMED, AND NICK TOOK ME OUT OFTEN TO BARS AND NIGHTCLUBS. I WAS NEVER ASKED FOR AN ID AND HE SEEMED TO KNOW EVERYONE ANYWAY. MY FAVORITE NIGHT OUT WAS IN NEW YORK WHEN WE WENT TO SEE BARRY WHITE AT RADIO CITY MUSIC HALL.
CITY
Music Hall RADIO CITY
BARRY WHITE
I HAD BEEN WORKING AT THE BRIGANTINE CASTLE PRIOR TO MEETING NICKY. IT WAS JUST BEFORE MY 15TH BIRTHDAY, AND AT THAT POINT, TO AVOID GETTING INTO TROUBLE, I COULDN'T TELL ANYONE MY TRUE AGE.
NICK THOUGHT I WAS 16, SO I BEGAN TO BELIEVE IT MYSELF. IT WAS AN EASY WHITE LIE UNTIL MY SWEET 16TH BIRTHDAY, WHEN I WANTED TO SHOW HIM OFF TO MY FRIENDS.
RANDEE
SANDRA
NICK
NICK, THERE'S SOMETHING YOU NEED TO KNOW ABOUT ME
NOTHING THAT YOU SAY EVER BOTHERS ME.
I'M ONLY 15. I'M GOING TO BE 16 VERY SOON. I WANT YOU TO KNOW SO YOU CAN CELEBRATE MY BIRTHDAY WITH ME. I'M SORRY I MISLED YOU, BUT WHEN I CAME FOR A JOB, I NEEDED TO BE 16 SO I HAD TO LIE. I NEVER KNEW THAT WE WOULD BECOME THIS CLOSE. I'M SO SORRY.
REALLY? YOU'RE ONLY 15?
FROM THAT MOMENT ON, WE WERE EVEN CLOSER. NICK WAS ABLE TO BE PART OF MY SPECIAL BIRTHDAY. AFTER THE FIRST YEAR OF DATING, I WAS ABLE TO GIVE UP MY VIRGINITY TO HIM WITHOUT GUILT AND FELT FORTUNATE MY FIRST LOVE UNDERSTOOD ABOUT THE DIFFERENCES IN MY BODY.
ONE DAY, I KNOCKED ON HIS APARTMENT DOOR.
UH... NICK'S SLEEPING. COME BACK LATER.
I JUST DROPPED BY... I'LL WAKE HIM UP.
LOOK, YOU DON'T WANT TO GO IN THERE RIGHT NOW, ALESIA. PLEASE UNDERSTAND.
ARE YOU OKAY?
GIVING UP MY VIRGINITY WAS SUCH A BIG THING! I TRUSTED EVERYTHING ABOUT HIM AND WANTED TO CONTINUE TO TRUST HIM AS OUR LOVE GREW.
NICK AND I MANAGED TO GET BACK TOGETHER FOR A SHORT TIME OVER THE NEXT YEAR, BUT THINGS WERE NEVER QUITE THE SAME. FIRST LOVE IS FIRST LOVE. I WAS WISER FOR THE NEXT RELATIONSHIP.

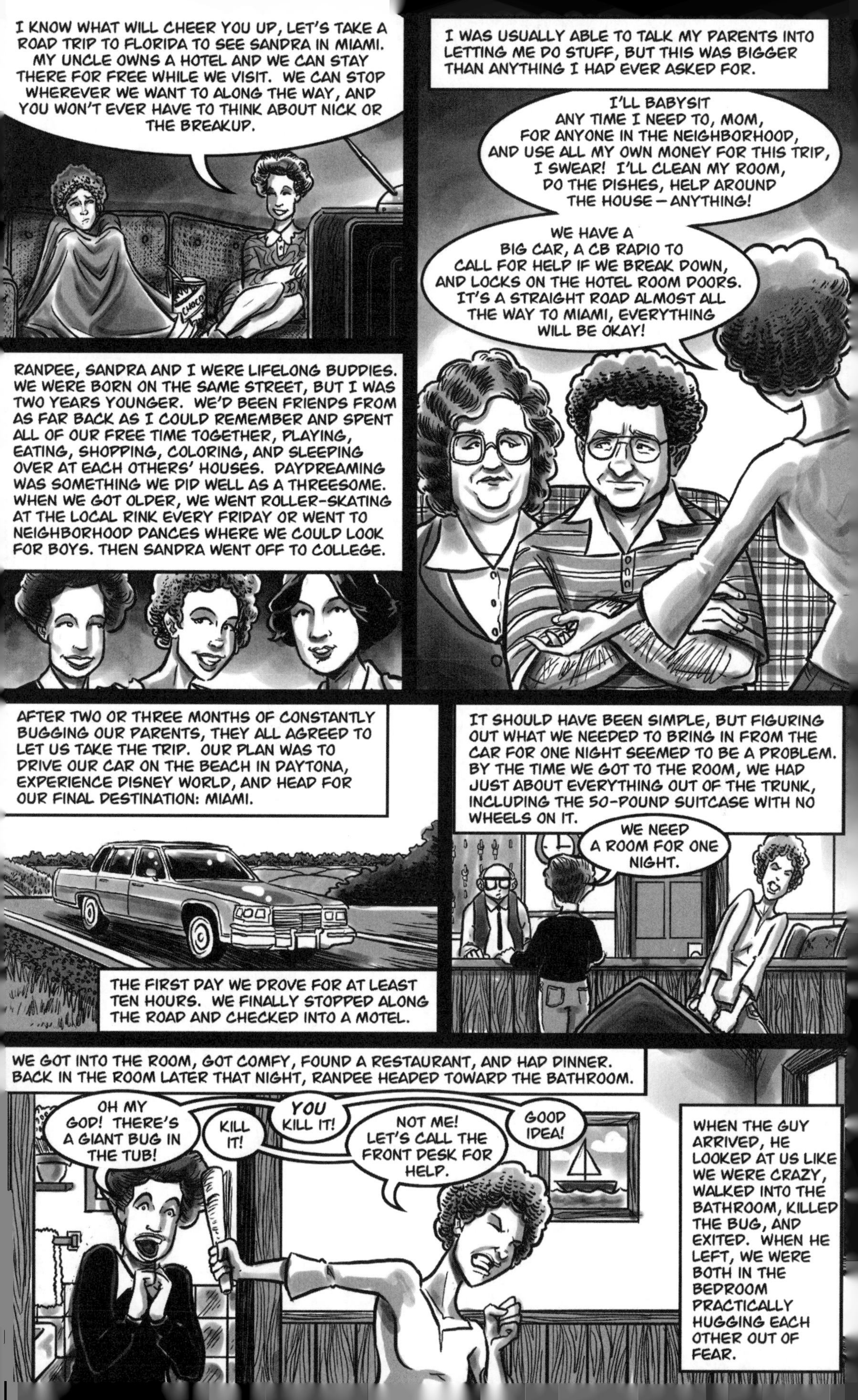

I KNOW WHAT WILL CHEER YOU UP, LET'S TAKE A ROAD TRIP TO FLORIDA TO SEE SANDRA IN MIAMI. MY UNCLE OWNS A HOTEL AND WE CAN STAY THERE FOR FREE WHILE WE VISIT. WE CAN STOP WHEREVER WE WANT TO ALONG THE WAY, AND YOU WON'T EVER HAVE TO THINK ABOUT NICK OR THE BREAKUP.
RANDEE, SANDRA AND I WERE LIFELONG BUDDIES. WE WERE BORN ON THE SAME STREET, BUT I WAS TWO YEARS YOUNGER. WE'D BEEN FRIENDS FROM AS FAR BACK AS I COULD REMEMBER AND SPENT ALL OF OUR FREE TIME TOGETHER, PLAYING, EATING, SHOPPING, COLORING, AND SLEEPING OVER AT EACH OTHERS' HOUSES. DAYDREAMING WAS SOMETHING WE DID WELL AS A THREESOME. WHEN WE GOT OLDER, WE WENT ROLLER-SKATING AT THE LOCAL RINK EVERY FRIDAY OR WENT TO NEIGHBORHOOD DANCES WHERE WE COULD LOOK FOR BOYS. THEN SANDRA WENT OFF TO COLLEGE.
I WAS USUALLY ABLE TO TALK MY PARENTS INTO LETTING ME DO STUFF, BUT THIS WAS BIGGER THAN ANYTHING I HAD EVER ASKED FOR.
I'LL BABYSIT ANY TIME I NEED TO, MOM, FOR ANYONE IN THE NEIGHBORHOOD, AND USE ALL MY OWN MONEY FOR THIS TRIP, I SWEAR! I'LL CLEAN MY ROOM, DO THE DISHES, HELP AROUND THE HOUSE – ANYTHING!
WE HAVE A BIG CAR, A CB RADIO TO CALL FOR HELP IF WE BREAK DOWN, AND LOCKS ON THE HOTEL ROOM DOORS. IT'S A STRAIGHT ROAD ALMOST ALL THE WAY TO MIAMI, EVERYTHING WILL BE OKAY!
AFTER TWO OR THREE MONTHS OF CONSTANTLY BUGGING OUR PARENTS, THEY ALL AGREED TO LET US TAKE THE TRIP. OUR PLAN WAS TO DRIVE OUR CAR ON THE BEACH IN DAYTONA, EXPERIENCE DISNEY WORLD, AND HEAD FOR OUR FINAL DESTINATION: MIAMI.
THE FIRST DAY WE DROVE FOR AT LEAST TEN HOURS. WE FINALLY STOPPED ALONG THE ROAD AND CHECKED INTO A MOTEL.
IT SHOULD HAVE BEEN SIMPLE, BUT FIGURING OUT WHAT WE NEEDED TO BRING IN FROM THE CAR FOR ONE NIGHT SEEMED TO BE A PROBLEM. BY THE TIME WE GOT TO THE ROOM, WE HAD JUST ABOUT EVERYTHING OUT OF THE TRUNK, INCLUDING THE 50-POUND SUITCASE WITH NO WHEELS ON IT.
WE NEED A ROOM FOR ONE NIGHT.
WE GOT INTO THE ROOM, GOT COMFY, FOUND A RESTAURANT, AND HAD DINNER. BACK IN THE ROOM LATER THAT NIGHT, RANDEE HEADED TOWARD THE BATHROOM.
OH MY GOD! THERE'S A GIANT BUG IN THE TUB!
KILL IT!
YOU KILL IT!
NOT ME! LET'S CALL THE FRONT DESK FOR HELP.
GOOD IDEA!
WHEN THE GUY ARRIVED, HE LOOKED AT US LIKE WE WERE CRAZY, WALKED INTO THE BATHROOM, KILLED THE BUG, AND EXITED. WHEN HE LEFT, WE WERE BOTH IN THE BEDROOM PRACTICALLY HUGGING EACH OTHER OUT OF FEAR.

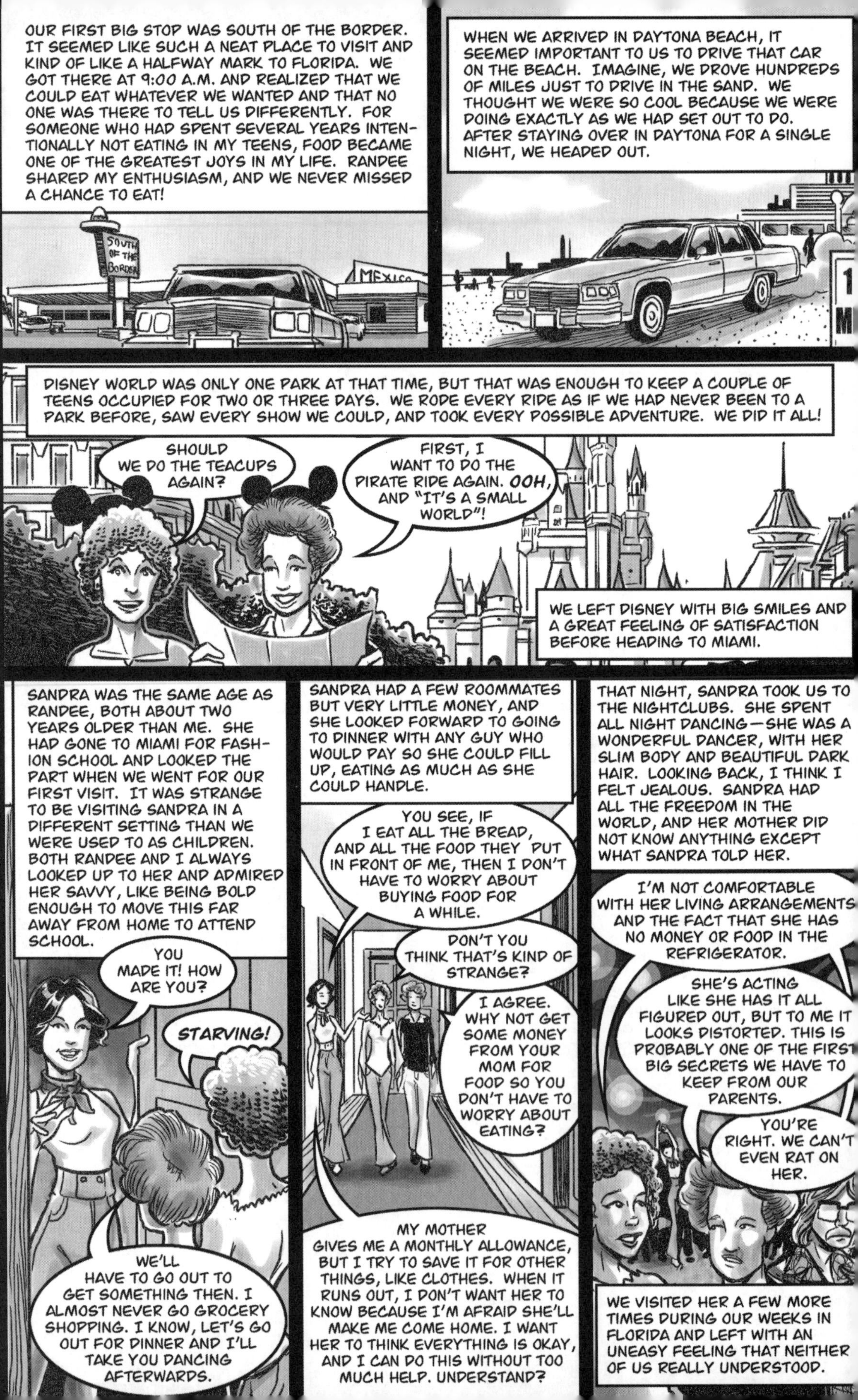
OUR FIRST BIG STOP WAS SOUTH OF THE BORDER. IT SEEMED LIKE SUCH A NEAT PLACE TO VISIT AND KIND OF LIKE A HALFWAY MARK TO FLORIDA. WE GOT THERE AT 9:00 A.M. AND REALIZED THAT WE COULD EAT WHATEVER WE WANTED AND THAT NO ONE WAS THERE TO TELL US DIFFERENTLY. FOR SOMEONE WHO HAD SPENT SEVERAL YEARS INTENTIONALLY NOT EATING IN MY TEENS, FOOD BECAME ONE OF THE GREATEST JOYS IN MY LIFE. RANDEE SHARED MY ENTHUSIASM, AND WE NEVER MISSED A CHANCE TO EAT!
SOUTH OF THE BORDER
MEXICO
WHEN WE ARRIVED IN DAYTONA BEACH, IT SEEMED IMPORTANT TO US TO DRIVE THAT CAR ON THE BEACH. IMAGINE, WE DROVE HUNDREDS OF MILES JUST TO DRIVE IN THE SAND. WE THOUGHT WE WERE SO COOL BECAUSE WE WERE DOING EXACTLY AS WE HAD SET OUT TO DO. AFTER STAYING OVER IN DAYTONA FOR A SINGLE NIGHT, WE HEADED OUT.
DISNEY WORLD WAS ONLY ONE PARK AT THAT TIME, BUT THAT WAS ENOUGH TO KEEP A COUPLE OF TEENS OCCUPIED FOR TWO OR THREE DAYS. WE RODE EVERY RIDE AS IF WE HAD NEVER BEEN TO A PARK BEFORE, SAW EVERY SHOW WE COULD, AND TOOK EVERY POSSIBLE ADVENTURE. WE DID IT ALL!
SHOULD WE DO THE TEACUPS AGAIN?
FIRST, I WANT TO DO THE PIRATE RIDE AGAIN. OOH, AND "IT'S A SMALL WORLD"!
WE LEFT DISNEY WITH BIG SMILES AND A GREAT FEELING OF SATISFACTION BEFORE HEADING TO MIAMI.
SANDRA WAS THE SAME AGE AS RANDEE, BOTH ABOUT TWO YEARS OLDER THAN ME. SHE HAD GONE TO MIAMI FOR FASHION SCHOOL AND LOOKED THE PART WHEN WE WENT FOR OUR FIRST VISIT. IT WAS STRANGE TO BE VISITING SANDRA IN A DIFFERENT SETTING THAN WE WERE USED TO AS CHILDREN. BOTH RANDEE AND I ALWAYS LOOKED UP TO HER AND ADMIRED HER SAVVY, LIKE BEING BOLD ENOUGH TO MOVE THIS FAR AWAY FROM HOME TO ATTEND SCHOOL.
YOU MADE IT! HOW ARE YOU?
STARVING!
WE'LL HAVE TO GO OUT TO GET SOMETHING THEN. I ALMOST NEVER GO GROCERY SHOPPING. I KNOW, LET'S GO OUT FOR DINNER AND I'LL TAKE YOU DANCING AFTERWARDS.
SANDRA HAD A FEW ROOMMATES BUT VERY LITTLE MONEY, AND SHE LOOKED FORWARD TO GOING TO DINNER WITH ANY GUY WHO WOULD PAY SO SHE COULD FILL UP, EATING AS MUCH AS SHE COULD HANDLE.
YOU SEE, IF I EAT ALL THE BREAD, AND ALL THE FOOD THEY PUT IN FRONT OF ME, THEN I DON'T HAVE TO WORRY ABOUT BUYING FOOD FOR A WHILE.
DON'T YOU THINK THAT'S KIND OF STRANGE?
I AGREE. WHY NOT GET SOME MONEY FROM YOUR MOM FOR FOOD SO YOU DON'T HAVE TO WORRY ABOUT EATING?
MY MOTHER GIVES ME A MONTHLY ALLOWANCE, BUT I TRY TO SAVE IT FOR OTHER THINGS, LIKE CLOTHES. WHEN IT RUNS OUT, I DON'T WANT HER TO KNOW BECAUSE I'M AFRAID SHE'LL MAKE ME COME HOME. I WANT HER TO THINK EVERYTHING IS OKAY, AND I CAN DO THIS WITHOUT TOO MUCH HELP. UNDERSTAND?
THAT NIGHT, SANDRA TOOK US TO THE NIGHTCLUBS. SHE SPENT ALL NIGHT DANCING—SHE WAS A WONDERFUL DANCER, WITH HER SLIM BODY AND BEAUTIFUL DARK HAIR. LOOKING BACK, I THINK I FELT JEALOUS. SANDRA HAD ALL THE FREEDOM IN THE WORLD, AND HER MOTHER DID NOT KNOW ANYTHING EXCEPT WHAT SANDRA TOLD HER.
I'M NOT COMFORTABLE WITH HER LIVING ARRANGEMENTS AND THE FACT THAT SHE HAS NO MONEY OR FOOD IN THE REFRIGERATOR.
SHE'S ACTING LIKE SHE HAS IT ALL FIGURED OUT, BUT TO ME IT LOOKS DISTORTED. THIS IS PROBABLY ONE OF THE FIRST BIG SECRETS WE HAVE TO KEEP FROM OUR PARENTS.
YOU'RE RIGHT. WE CAN'T EVEN RAT ON HER.
WE VISITED HER A FEW MORE TIMES DURING OUR WEEKS IN FLORIDA AND LEFT WITH AN UNEASY FEELING THAT NEITHER OF US REALLY UNDERSTOOD.

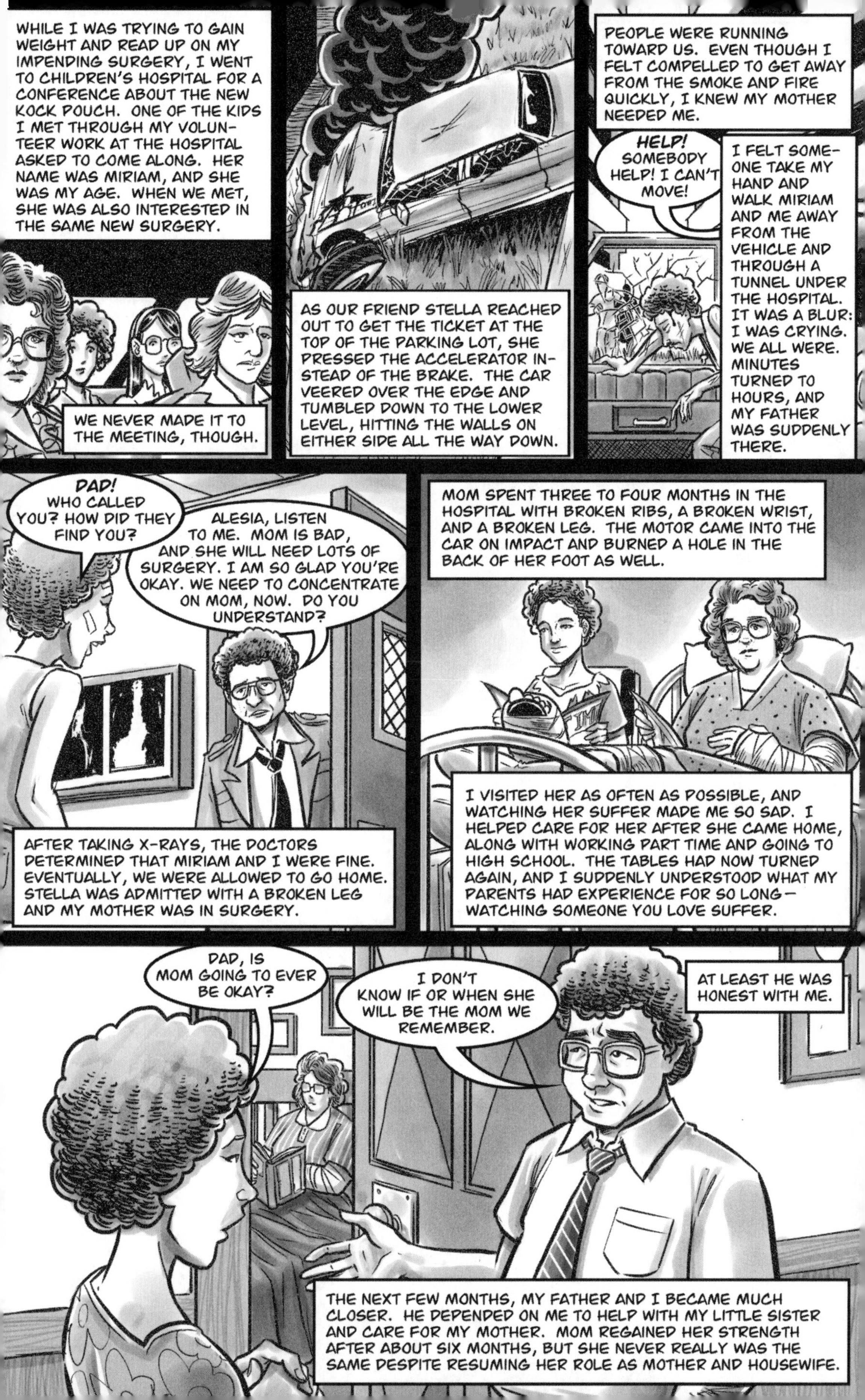
WHILE I WAS TRYING TO GAIN WEIGHT AND READ UP ON MY IMPENDING SURGERY, I WENT TO CHILDREN'S HOSPITAL FOR A CONFERENCE ABOUT THE NEW KOCK POUCH. ONE OF THE KIDS I MET THROUGH MY VOLUNTEER WORK AT THE HOSPITAL ASKED TO COME ALONG. HER NAME WAS MIRIAM, AND SHE WAS MY AGE. WHEN WE MET, SHE WAS ALSO INTERESTED IN THE SAME NEW SURGERY.
WE NEVER MADE IT TO THE MEETING, THOUGH.
AS OUR FRIEND STELLA REACHED OUT TO GET THE TICKET AT THE TOP OF THE PARKING LOT, SHE PRESSED THE ACCELERATOR INSTEAD OF THE BRAKE. THE CAR VEERED OVER THE EDGE AND TUMBLED DOWN TO THE LOWER LEVEL, HITTING THE WALLS ON EITHER SIDE ALL THE WAY DOWN.
PEOPLE WERE RUNNING TOWARD US. EVEN THOUGH I FELT COMPELLED TO GET AWAY FROM THE SMOKE AND FIRE QUICKLY, I KNEW MY MOTHER NEEDED ME.
HELP! SOMEBODY HELP! I CAN'T MOVE!
I FELT SOMEONE TAKE MY HAND AND WALK MIRIAM AND ME AWAY FROM THE VEHICLE AND THROUGH A TUNNEL UNDER THE HOSPITAL. IT WAS A BLUR: I WAS CRYING. WE ALL WERE. MINUTES TURNED TO HOURS, AND MY FATHER WAS SUDDENLY THERE.
DAD! WHO CALLED YOU? HOW DID THEY FIND YOU?
ALESIA, LISTEN TO ME. MOM IS BAD, AND SHE WILL NEED LOTS OF SURGERY. I AM SO GLAD YOU'RE OKAY. WE NEED TO CONCENTRATE ON MOM, NOW. DO YOU UNDERSTAND?
AFTER TAKING X-RAYS, THE DOCTORS DETERMINED THAT MIRIAM AND I WERE FINE. EVENTUALLY, WE WERE ALLOWED TO GO HOME. STELLA WAS ADMITTED WITH A BROKEN LEG AND MY MOTHER WAS IN SURGERY.
MOM SPENT THREE TO FOUR MONTHS IN THE HOSPITAL WITH BROKEN RIBS, A BROKEN WRIST, AND A BROKEN LEG. THE MOTOR CAME INTO THE CAR ON IMPACT AND BURNED A HOLE IN THE BACK OF HER FOOT AS WELL.
I VISITED HER AS OFTEN AS POSSIBLE, AND WATCHING HER SUFFER MADE ME SO SAD. I HELPED CARE FOR HER AFTER SHE CAME HOME, ALONG WITH WORKING PART TIME AND GOING TO HIGH SCHOOL. THE TABLES HAD NOW TURNED AGAIN, AND I SUDDENLY UNDERSTOOD WHAT MY PARENTS HAD EXPERIENCE FOR SO LONG—WATCHING SOMEONE YOU LOVE SUFFER.
DAD, IS MOM GOING TO EVER BE OKAY?
I DON'T KNOW IF OR WHEN SHE WILL BE THE MOM WE REMEMBER.
AT LEAST HE WAS HONEST WITH ME.
THE NEXT FEW MONTHS, MY FATHER AND I BECAME MUCH CLOSER. HE DEPENDED ON ME TO HELP WITH MY LITTLE SISTER AND CARE FOR MY MOTHER. MOM REGAINED HER STRENGTH AFTER ABOUT SIX MONTHS, BUT SHE NEVER REALLY WAS THE SAME DESPITE RESUMING HER ROLE AS MOTHER AND HOUSEWIFE.

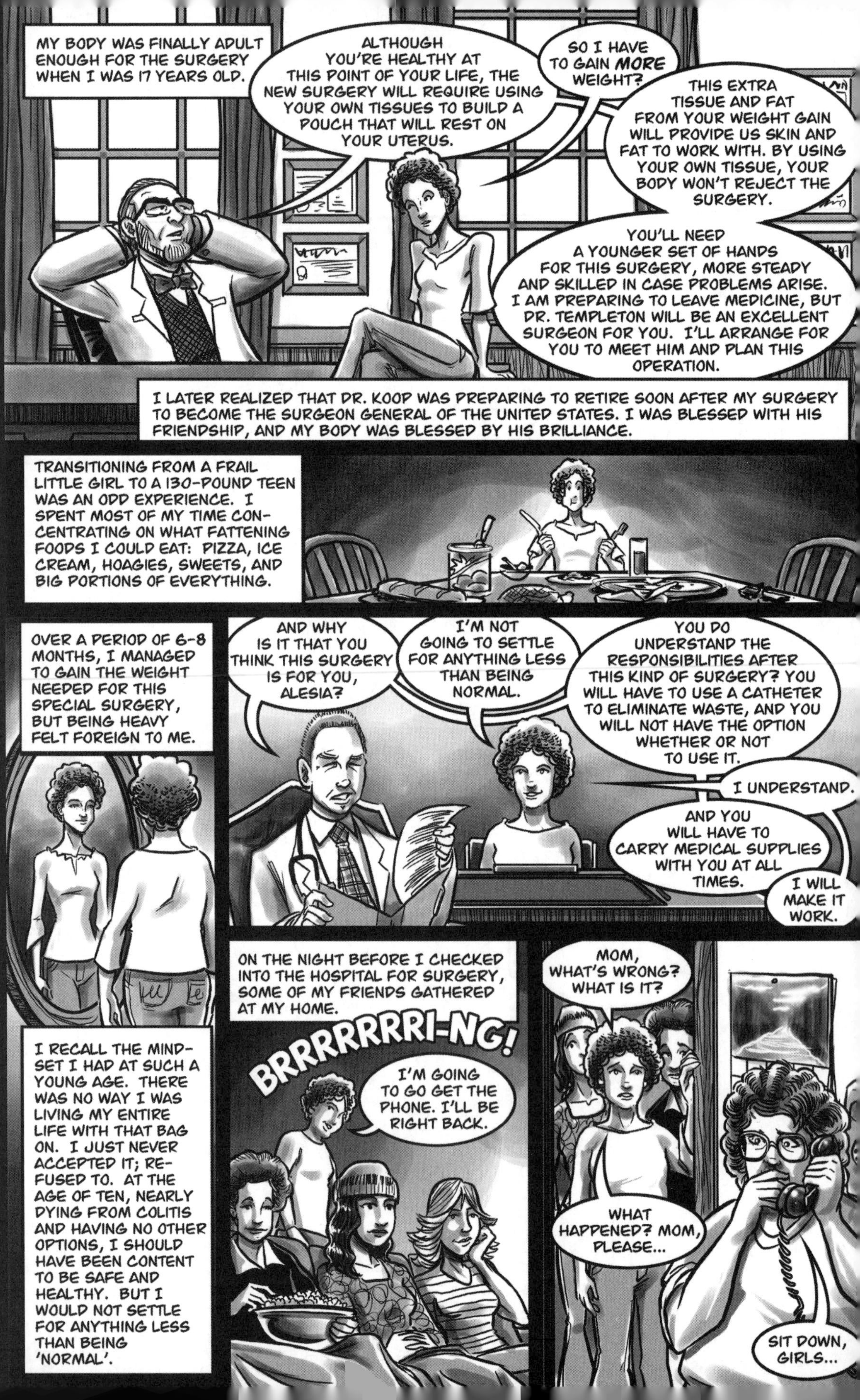
MY BODY WAS FINALLY ADULT ENOUGH FOR THE SURGERY WHEN I WAS 17 YEARS OLD.
ALTHOUGH YOU'RE HEALTHY AT THIS POINT OF YOUR LIFE, THE NEW SURGERY WILL REQUIRE USING YOUR OWN TISSUES TO BUILD A POUCH THAT WILL REST ON YOUR UTERUS.
SO I HAVE TO GAIN **MORE** WEIGHT?
THIS EXTRA TISSUE AND FAT FROM YOUR WEIGHT GAIN WILL PROVIDE US SKIN AND FAT TO WORK WITH. BY USING YOUR OWN TISSUE, YOUR BODY WON'T REJECT THE SURGERY.
YOU'LL NEED A YOUNGER SET OF HANDS FOR THIS SURGERY, MORE STEADY AND SKILLED IN CASE PROBLEMS ARISE. I AM PREPARING TO LEAVE MEDICINE, BUT DR. TEMPLETON WILL BE AN EXCELLENT SURGEON FOR YOU. I'LL ARRANGE FOR YOU TO MEET HIM AND PLAN THIS OPERATION.
I LATER REALIZED THAT DR. KOOP WAS PREPARING TO RETIRE SOON AFTER MY SURGERY TO BECOME THE SURGEON GENERAL OF THE UNITED STATES. I WAS BLESSED WITH HIS FRIENDSHIP, AND MY BODY WAS BLESSED BY HIS BRILLIANCE.
TRANSITIONING FROM A FRAIL LITTLE GIRL TO A 130-POUND TEEN WAS AN ODD EXPERIENCE. I SPENT MOST OF MY TIME CONCENTRATING ON WHAT FATTENING FOODS I COULD EAT: PIZZA, ICE CREAM, HOAGIES, SWEETS, AND BIG PORTIONS OF EVERYTHING.
OVER A PERIOD OF 6–8 MONTHS, I MANAGED TO GAIN THE WEIGHT NEEDED FOR THIS SPECIAL SURGERY, BUT BEING HEAVY FELT FOREIGN TO ME.
AND WHY IS IT THAT YOU THINK THIS SURGERY IS FOR YOU, ALESIA?
I'M NOT GOING TO SETTLE FOR ANYTHING LESS THAN BEING NORMAL.
YOU DO UNDERSTAND THE RESPONSIBILITIES AFTER THIS KIND OF SURGERY? YOU WILL HAVE TO USE A CATHETER TO ELIMINATE WASTE, AND YOU WILL NOT HAVE THE OPTION WHETHER OR NOT TO USE IT.
I UNDERSTAND.
AND YOU WILL HAVE TO CARRY MEDICAL SUPPLIES WITH YOU AT ALL TIMES.
I WILL MAKE IT WORK.
I RECALL THE MINDSET I HAD AT SUCH A YOUNG AGE. THERE WAS NO WAY I WAS LIVING MY ENTIRE LIFE WITH THAT BAG ON. I JUST NEVER ACCEPTED IT; REFUSED TO. AT THE AGE OF TEN, NEARLY DYING FROM COLITIS AND HAVING NO OTHER OPTIONS, I SHOULD HAVE BEEN CONTENT TO BE SAFE AND HEALTHY. BUT I WOULD NOT SETTLE FOR ANYTHING LESS THAN BEING 'NORMAL'.
ON THE NIGHT BEFORE I CHECKED INTO THE HOSPITAL FOR SURGERY, SOME OF MY FRIENDS GATHERED AT MY HOME.
BRRRRRRRI-NG!
I'M GOING TO GO GET THE PHONE. I'LL BE RIGHT BACK.
MOM, WHAT'S WRONG? WHAT IS IT?
WHAT HAPPENED? MOM, PLEASE...
SIT DOWN, GIRLS...

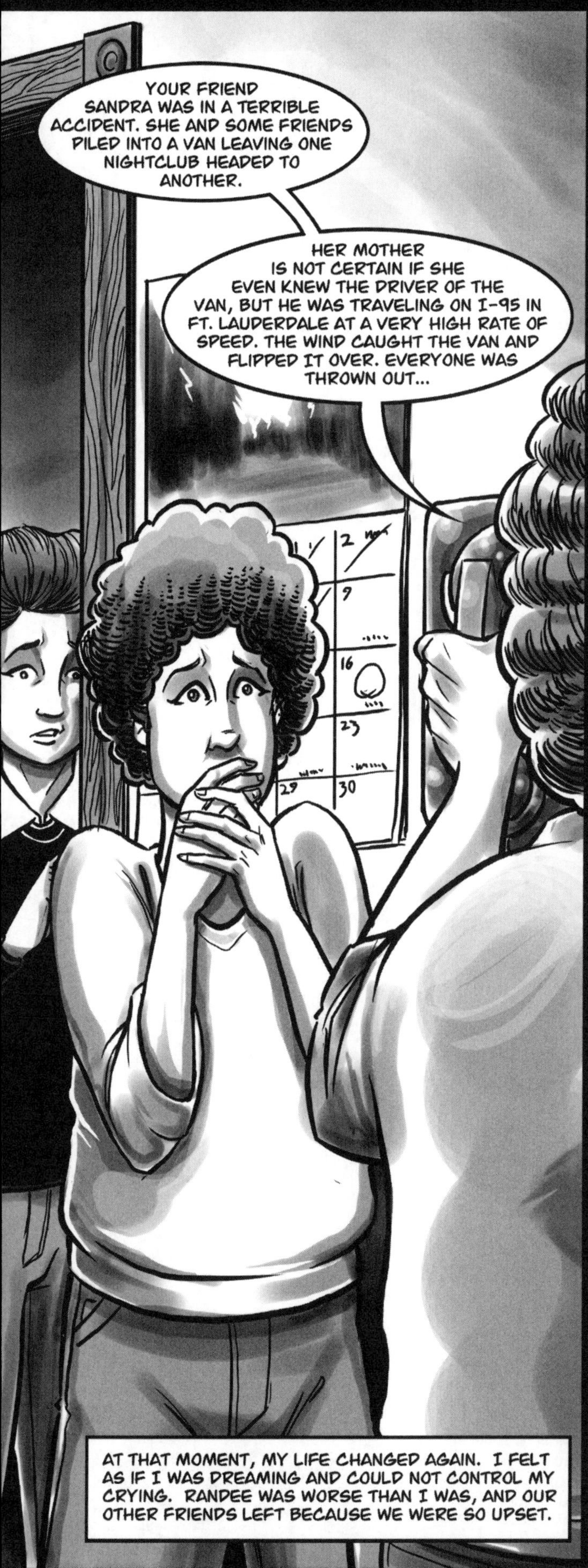
YOUR FRIEND SANDRA WAS IN A TERRIBLE ACCIDENT. SHE AND SOME FRIENDS PILED INTO A VAN LEAVING ONE NIGHTCLUB HEADED TO ANOTHER.
HER MOTHER IS NOT CERTAIN IF SHE EVEN KNEW THE DRIVER OF THE VAN, BUT HE WAS TRAVELING ON I-95 IN FT. LAUDERDALE AT A VERY HIGH RATE OF SPEED. THE WIND CAUGHT THE VAN AND FLIPPED IT OVER. EVERYONE WAS THROWN OUT...
AT THAT MOMENT, MY LIFE CHANGED AGAIN. I FELT AS IF I WAS DREAMING AND COULD NOT CONTROL MY CRYING. RANDEE WAS WORSE THAN I WAS, AND OUR OTHER FRIENDS LEFT BECAUSE WE WERE SO UPSET.

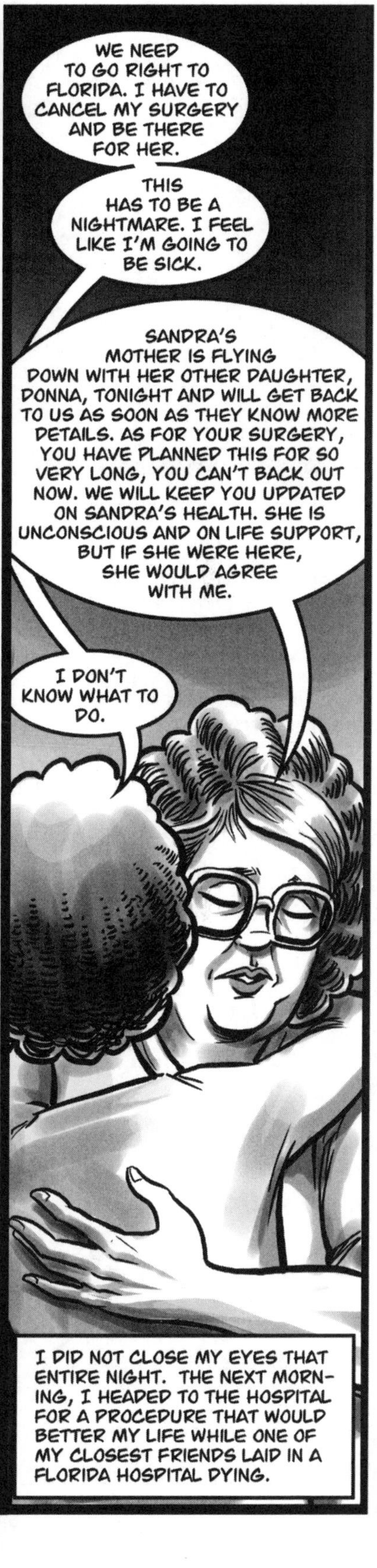
WE NEED TO GO RIGHT TO FLORIDA. I HAVE TO CANCEL MY SURGERY AND BE THERE FOR HER.
THIS HAS TO BE A NIGHTMARE. I FEEL LIKE I'M GOING TO BE SICK.
SANDRA'S MOTHER IS FLYING DOWN WITH HER OTHER DAUGHTER, DONNA, TONIGHT AND WILL GET BACK TO US AS SOON AS THEY KNOW MORE DETAILS. AS FOR YOUR SURGERY, YOU HAVE PLANNED THIS FOR SO VERY LONG, YOU CAN'T BACK OUT NOW. WE WILL KEEP YOU UPDATED ON SANDRA'S HEALTH. SHE IS UNCONSCIOUS AND ON LIFE SUPPORT, BUT IF SHE WERE HERE, SHE WOULD AGREE WITH ME.
I DON'T KNOW WHAT TO DO.
I DID NOT CLOSE MY EYES THAT ENTIRE NIGHT. THE NEXT MORNING, I HEADED TO THE HOSPITAL FOR A PROCEDURE THAT WOULD BETTER MY LIFE WHILE ONE OF MY CLOSEST FRIENDS LAID IN A FLORIDA HOSPITAL DYING.

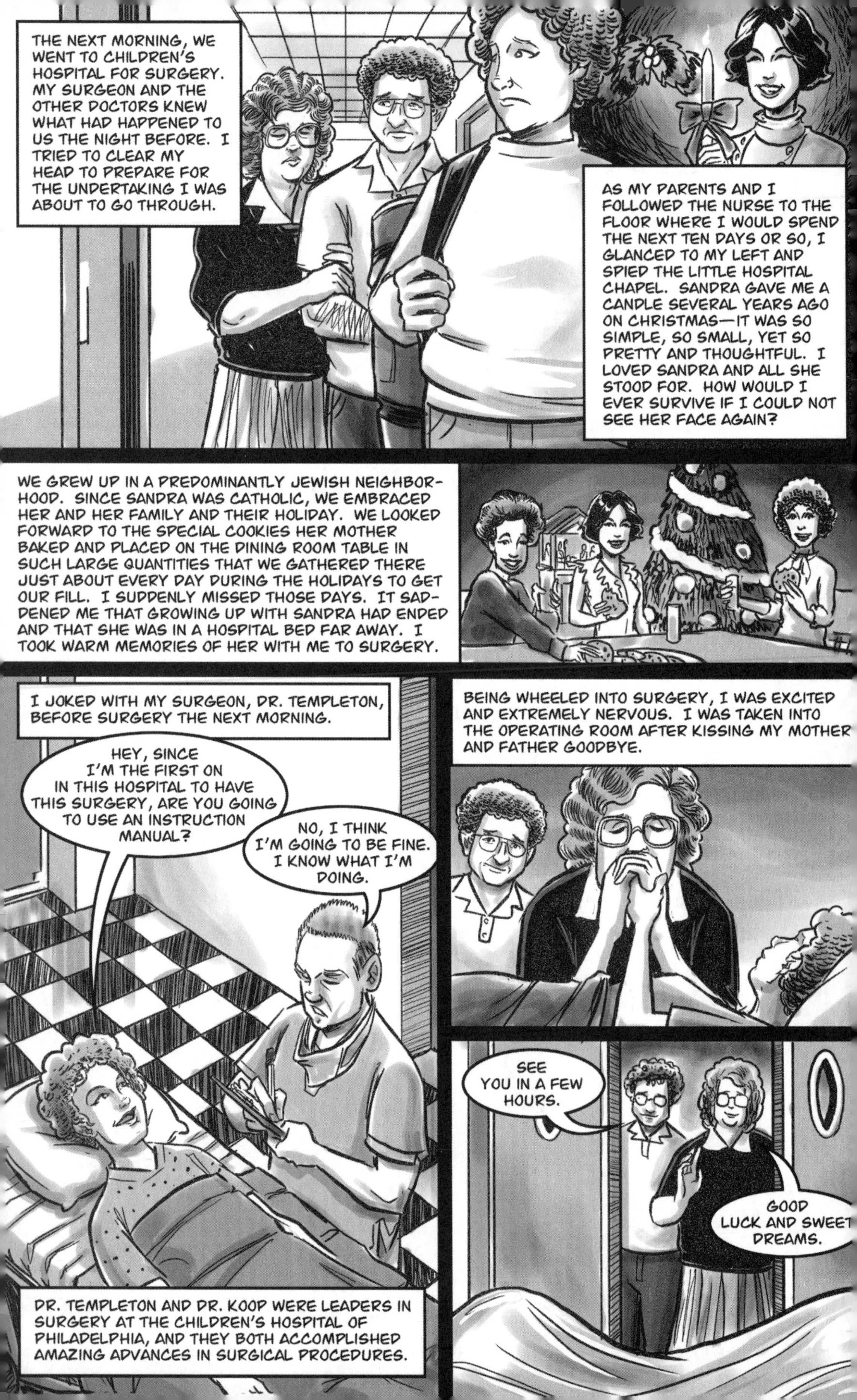
THE NEXT MORNING, WE WENT TO CHILDREN'S HOSPITAL FOR SURGERY. MY SURGEON AND THE OTHER DOCTORS KNEW WHAT HAD HAPPENED TO US THE NIGHT BEFORE. I TRIED TO CLEAR MY HEAD TO PREPARE FOR THE UNDERTAKING I WAS ABOUT TO GO THROUGH.
AS MY PARENTS AND I FOLLOWED THE NURSE TO THE FLOOR WHERE I WOULD SPEND THE NEXT TEN DAYS OR SO, I GLANCED TO MY LEFT AND SPIED THE LITTLE HOSPITAL CHAPEL. SANDRA GAVE ME A CANDLE SEVERAL YEARS AGO ON CHRISTMAS—IT WAS SO SIMPLE, SO SMALL, YET SO PRETTY AND THOUGHTFUL. I LOVED SANDRA AND ALL SHE STOOD FOR. HOW WOULD I EVER SURVIVE IF I COULD NOT SEE HER FACE AGAIN?
WE GREW UP IN A PREDOMINANTLY JEWISH NEIGHBORHOOD. SINCE SANDRA WAS CATHOLIC, WE EMBRACED HER AND HER FAMILY AND THEIR HOLIDAY. WE LOOKED FORWARD TO THE SPECIAL COOKIES HER MOTHER BAKED AND PLACED ON THE DINING ROOM TABLE IN SUCH LARGE QUANTITIES THAT WE GATHERED THERE JUST ABOUT EVERY DAY DURING THE HOLIDAYS TO GET OUR FILL. I SUDDENLY MISSED THOSE DAYS. IT SADDENED ME THAT GROWING UP WITH SANDRA HAD ENDED AND THAT SHE WAS IN A HOSPITAL BED FAR AWAY. I TOOK WARM MEMORIES OF HER WITH ME TO SURGERY.
I JOKED WITH MY SURGEON, DR. TEMPLETON, BEFORE SURGERY THE NEXT MORNING.
HEY, SINCE I'M THE FIRST ON IN THIS HOSPITAL TO HAVE THIS SURGERY, ARE YOU GOING TO USE AN INSTRUCTION MANUAL?
NO, I THINK I'M GOING TO BE FINE. I KNOW WHAT I'M DOING.
DR. TEMPLETON AND DR. KOOP WERE LEADERS IN SURGERY AT THE CHILDREN'S HOSPITAL OF PHILADELPHIA, AND THEY BOTH ACCOMPLISHED AMAZING ADVANCES IN SURGICAL PROCEDURES.
BEING WHEELED INTO SURGERY, I WAS EXCITED AND EXTREMELY NERVOUS. I WAS TAKEN INTO THE OPERATING ROOM AFTER KISSING MY MOTHER AND FATHER GOODBYE.
SEE YOU IN A FEW HOURS.
GOOD LUCK AND SWEET DREAMS.

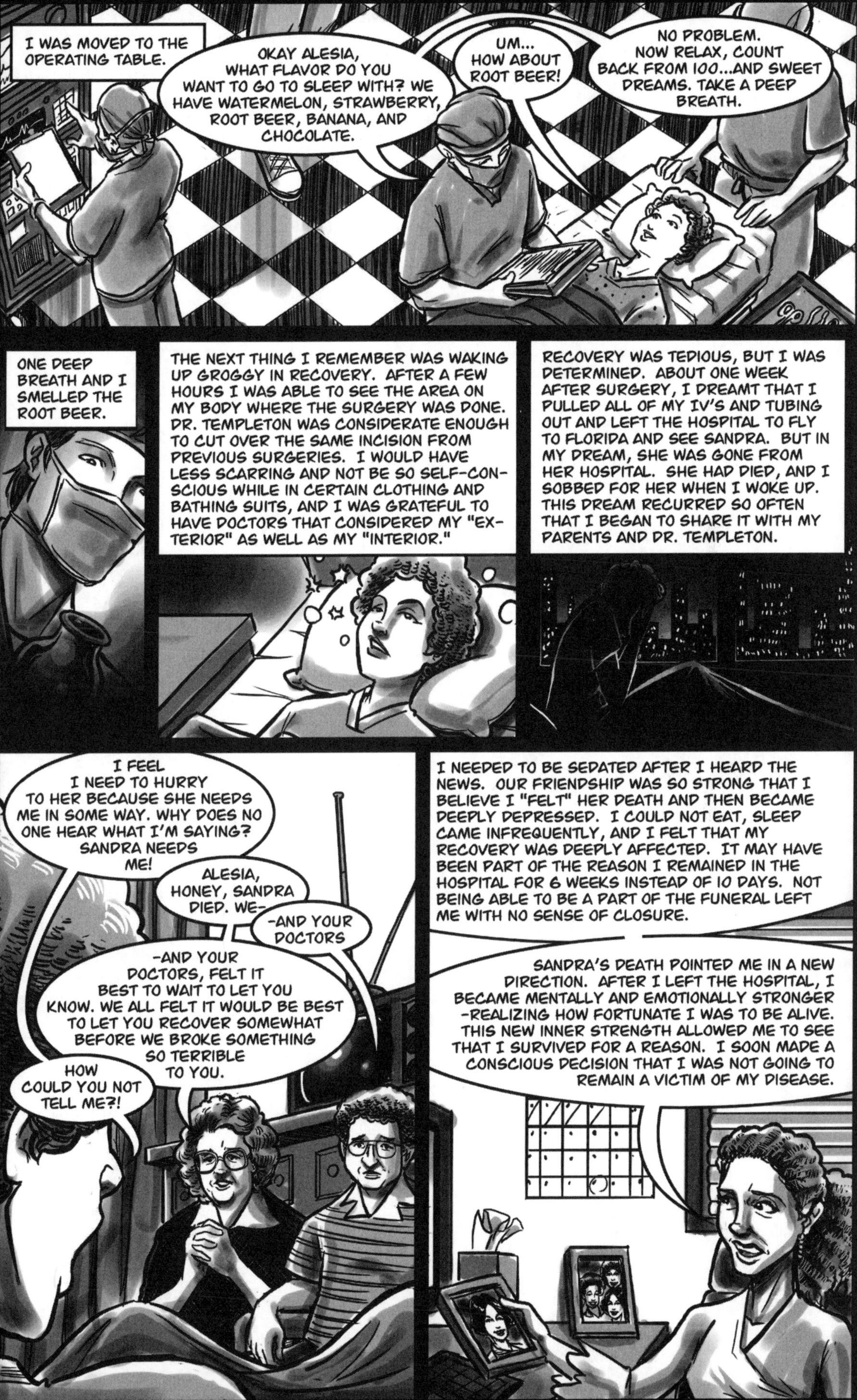
I WAS MOVED TO THE OPERATING TABLE.
OKAY ALESIA, WHAT FLAVOR DO YOU WANT TO GO TO SLEEP WITH? WE HAVE WATERMELON, STRAWBERRY, ROOT BEER, BANANA, AND CHOCOLATE.
UM... HOW ABOUT ROOT BEER!
NO PROBLEM. NOW RELAX, COUNT BACK FROM 100...AND SWEET DREAMS. TAKE A DEEP BREATH.
ONE DEEP BREATH AND I SMELLED THE ROOT BEER.
THE NEXT THING I REMEMBER WAS WAKING UP GROGGY IN RECOVERY. AFTER A FEW HOURS I WAS ABLE TO SEE THE AREA ON MY BODY WHERE THE SURGERY WAS DONE. DR. TEMPLETON WAS CONSIDERATE ENOUGH TO CUT OVER THE SAME INCISION FROM PREVIOUS SURGERIES. I WOULD HAVE LESS SCARRING AND NOT BE SO SELF-CONSCIOUS WHILE IN CERTAIN CLOTHING AND BATHING SUITS, AND I WAS GRATEFUL TO HAVE DOCTORS THAT CONSIDERED MY "EXTERIOR" AS WELL AS MY "INTERIOR."
RECOVERY WAS TEDIOUS, BUT I WAS DETERMINED. ABOUT ONE WEEK AFTER SURGERY, I DREAMT THAT I PULLED ALL OF MY IV'S AND TUBING OUT AND LEFT THE HOSPITAL TO FLY TO FLORIDA AND SEE SANDRA. BUT IN MY DREAM, SHE WAS GONE FROM HER HOSPITAL. SHE HAD DIED, AND I SOBBED FOR HER WHEN I WOKE UP. THIS DREAM RECURRED SO OFTEN THAT I BEGAN TO SHARE IT WITH MY PARENTS AND DR. TEMPLETON.
I FEEL I NEED TO HURRY TO HER BECAUSE SHE NEEDS ME IN SOME WAY. WHY DOES NO ONE HEAR WHAT I'M SAYING? SANDRA NEEDS ME!
ALESIA, HONEY, SANDRA DIED. WE-
-AND YOUR DOCTORS
-AND YOUR DOCTORS, FELT IT BEST TO WAIT TO LET YOU KNOW. WE ALL FELT IT WOULD BE BEST TO LET YOU RECOVER SOMEWHAT BEFORE WE BROKE SOMETHING SO TERRIBLE TO YOU.
HOW COULD YOU NOT TELL ME?!
I NEEDED TO BE SEDATED AFTER I HEARD THE NEWS. OUR FRIENDSHIP WAS SO STRONG THAT I BELIEVE I "FELT" HER DEATH AND THEN BECAME DEEPLY DEPRESSED. I COULD NOT EAT, SLEEP CAME INFREQUENTLY, AND I FELT THAT MY RECOVERY WAS DEEPLY AFFECTED. IT MAY HAVE BEEN PART OF THE REASON I REMAINED IN THE HOSPITAL FOR 6 WEEKS INSTEAD OF 10 DAYS. NOT BEING ABLE TO BE A PART OF THE FUNERAL LEFT ME WITH NO SENSE OF CLOSURE.
SANDRA'S DEATH POINTED ME IN A NEW DIRECTION. AFTER I LEFT THE HOSPITAL, I BECAME MENTALLY AND EMOTIONALLY STRONGER -REALIZING HOW FORTUNATE I WAS TO BE ALIVE. THIS NEW INNER STRENGTH ALLOWED ME TO SEE THAT I SURVIVED FOR A REASON. I SOON MADE A CONSCIOUS DECISION THAT I WAS NOT GOING TO REMAIN A VICTIM OF MY DISEASE.

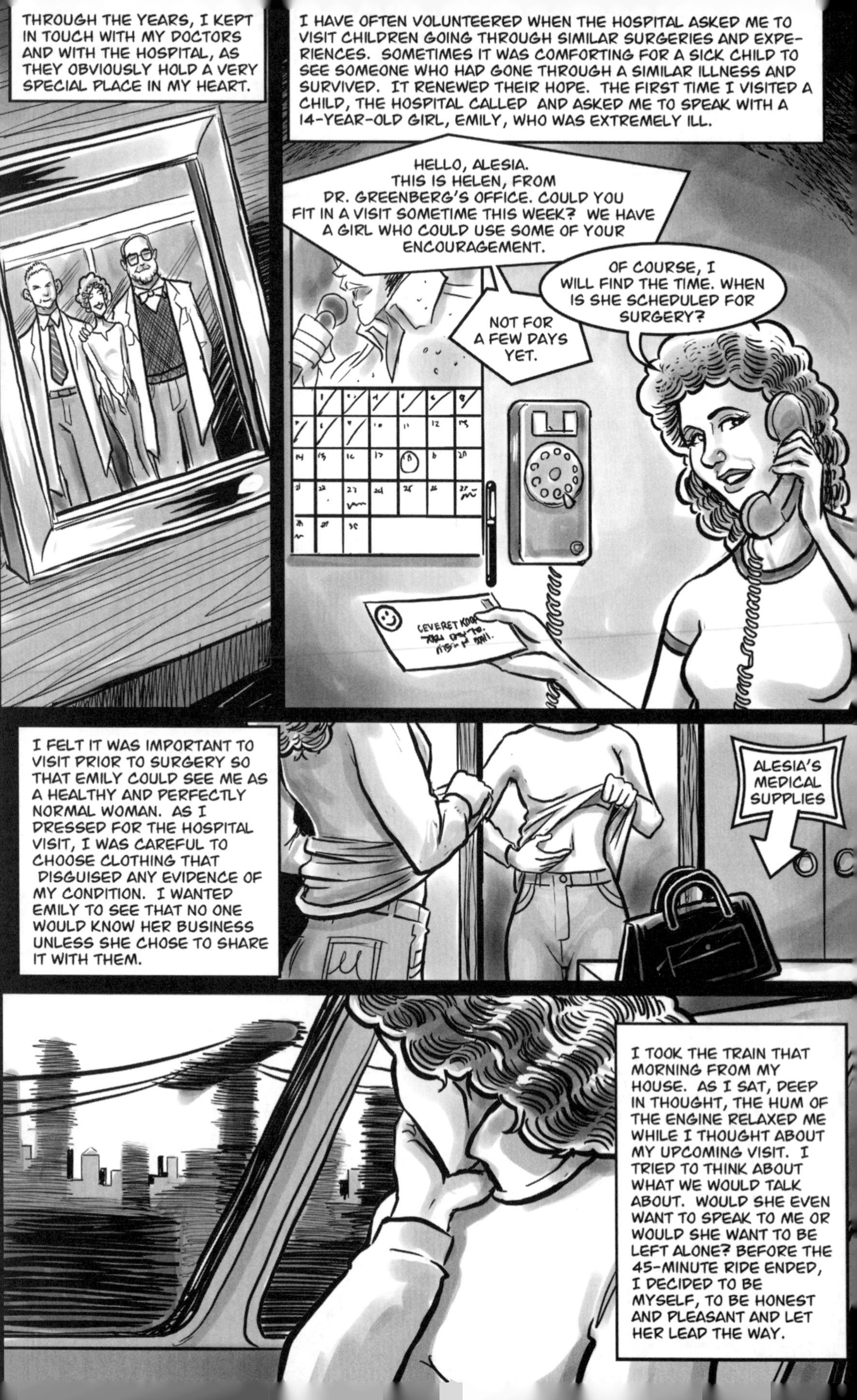
THROUGH THE YEARS, I KEPT IN TOUCH WITH MY DOCTORS AND WITH THE HOSPITAL, AS THEY OBVIOUSLY HOLD A VERY SPECIAL PLACE IN MY HEART.
I HAVE OFTEN VOLUNTEERED WHEN THE HOSPITAL ASKED ME TO VISIT CHILDREN GOING THROUGH SIMILAR SURGERIES AND EXPERIENCES. SOMETIMES IT WAS COMFORTING FOR A SICK CHILD TO SEE SOMEONE WHO HAD GONE THROUGH A SIMILAR ILLNESS AND SURVIVED. IT RENEWED THEIR HOPE. THE FIRST TIME I VISITED A CHILD, THE HOSPITAL CALLED AND ASKED ME TO SPEAK WITH A 14-YEAR-OLD GIRL, EMILY, WHO WAS EXTREMELY ILL.
HELLO, ALESIA. THIS IS HELEN, FROM DR. GREENBERG'S OFFICE. COULD YOU FIT IN A VISIT SOMETIME THIS WEEK? WE HAVE A GIRL WHO COULD USE SOME OF YOUR ENCOURAGEMENT.
OF COURSE, I WILL FIND THE TIME. WHEN IS SHE SCHEDULED FOR SURGERY?
NOT FOR A FEW DAYS YET.
I FELT IT WAS IMPORTANT TO VISIT PRIOR TO SURGERY SO THAT EMILY COULD SEE ME AS A HEALTHY AND PERFECTLY NORMAL WOMAN. AS I DRESSED FOR THE HOSPITAL VISIT, I WAS CAREFUL TO CHOOSE CLOTHING THAT DISGUISED ANY EVIDENCE OF MY CONDITION. I WANTED EMILY TO SEE THAT NO ONE WOULD KNOW HER BUSINESS UNLESS SHE CHOSE TO SHARE IT WITH THEM.
ALESIA'S MEDICAL SUPPLIES
I TOOK THE TRAIN THAT MORNING FROM MY HOUSE. AS I SAT, DEEP IN THOUGHT, THE HUM OF THE ENGINE RELAXED ME WHILE I THOUGHT ABOUT MY UPCOMING VISIT. I TRIED TO THINK ABOUT WHAT WE WOULD TALK ABOUT. WOULD SHE EVEN WANT TO SPEAK TO ME OR WOULD SHE WANT TO BE LEFT ALONE? BEFORE THE 45-MINUTE RIDE ENDED, I DECIDED TO BE MYSELF, TO BE HONEST AND PLEASANT AND LET HER LEAD THE WAY.

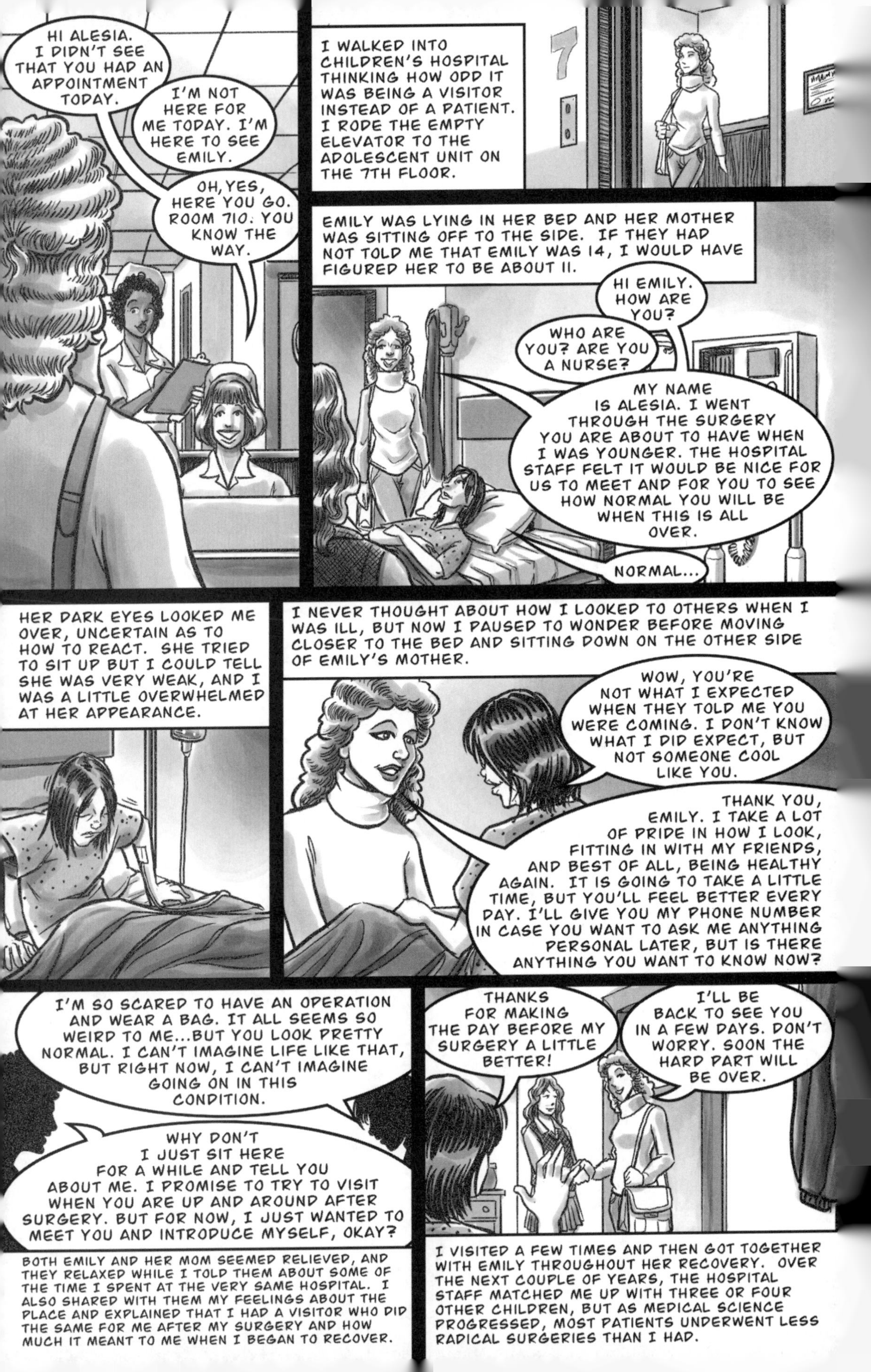
HI ALESIA. I DIDN'T SEE THAT YOU HAD AN APPOINTMENT TODAY.
I'M NOT HERE FOR ME TODAY. I'M HERE TO SEE EMILY.
OH, YES, HERE YOU GO. ROOM 710. YOU KNOW THE WAY.
I WALKED INTO CHILDREN'S HOSPITAL THINKING HOW ODD IT WAS BEING A VISITOR INSTEAD OF A PATIENT. I RODE THE EMPTY ELEVATOR TO THE ADOLESCENT UNIT ON THE 7TH FLOOR.
7
EMILY WAS LYING IN HER BED AND HER MOTHER WAS SITTING OFF TO THE SIDE. IF THEY HAD NOT TOLD ME THAT EMILY WAS 14, I WOULD HAVE FIGURED HER TO BE ABOUT 11.
HI EMILY. HOW ARE YOU?
WHO ARE YOU? ARE YOU A NURSE?
MY NAME IS ALESIA. I WENT THROUGH THE SURGERY YOU ARE ABOUT TO HAVE WHEN I WAS YOUNGER. THE HOSPITAL STAFF FELT IT WOULD BE NICE FOR US TO MEET AND FOR YOU TO SEE HOW NORMAL YOU WILL BE WHEN THIS IS ALL OVER.
NORMAL...
HER DARK EYES LOOKED ME OVER, UNCERTAIN AS TO HOW TO REACT. SHE TRIED TO SIT UP BUT I COULD TELL SHE WAS VERY WEAK, AND I WAS A LITTLE OVERWHELMED AT HER APPEARANCE.
I NEVER THOUGHT ABOUT HOW I LOOKED TO OTHERS WHEN I WAS ILL, BUT NOW I PAUSED TO WONDER BEFORE MOVING CLOSER TO THE BED AND SITTING DOWN ON THE OTHER SIDE OF EMILY'S MOTHER.
WOW, YOU'RE NOT WHAT I EXPECTED WHEN THEY TOLD ME YOU WERE COMING. I DON'T KNOW WHAT I DID EXPECT, BUT NOT SOMEONE COOL LIKE YOU.
THANK YOU, EMILY. I TAKE A LOT OF PRIDE IN HOW I LOOK, FITTING IN WITH MY FRIENDS, AND BEST OF ALL, BEING HEALTHY AGAIN. IT IS GOING TO TAKE A LITTLE TIME, BUT YOU'LL FEEL BETTER EVERY DAY. I'LL GIVE YOU MY PHONE NUMBER IN CASE YOU WANT TO ASK ME ANYTHING PERSONAL LATER, BUT IS THERE ANYTHING YOU WANT TO KNOW NOW?
I'M SO SCARED TO HAVE AN OPERATION AND WEAR A BAG. IT ALL SEEMS SO WEIRD TO ME...BUT YOU LOOK PRETTY NORMAL. I CAN'T IMAGINE LIFE LIKE THAT, BUT RIGHT NOW, I CAN'T IMAGINE GOING ON IN THIS CONDITION.
WHY DON'T I JUST SIT HERE FOR A WHILE AND TELL YOU ABOUT ME. I PROMISE TO TRY TO VISIT WHEN YOU ARE UP AND AROUND AFTER SURGERY. BUT FOR NOW, I JUST WANTED TO MEET YOU AND INTRODUCE MYSELF, OKAY?
BOTH EMILY AND HER MOM SEEMED RELIEVED, AND THEY RELAXED WHILE I TOLD THEM ABOUT SOME OF THE TIME I SPENT AT THE VERY SAME HOSPITAL. I ALSO SHARED WITH THEM MY FEELINGS ABOUT THE PLACE AND EXPLAINED THAT I HAD A VISITOR WHO DID THE SAME FOR ME AFTER MY SURGERY AND HOW MUCH IT MEANT TO ME WHEN I BEGAN TO RECOVER.
THANKS FOR MAKING THE DAY BEFORE MY SURGERY A LITTLE BETTER!
I'LL BE BACK TO SEE YOU IN A FEW DAYS. DON'T WORRY. SOON THE HARD PART WILL BE OVER.
I VISITED A FEW TIMES AND THEN GOT TOGETHER WITH EMILY THROUGHOUT HER RECOVERY. OVER THE NEXT COUPLE OF YEARS, THE HOSPITAL STAFF MATCHED ME UP WITH THREE OR FOUR OTHER CHILDREN, BUT AS MEDICAL SCIENCE PROGRESSED, MOST PATIENTS UNDERWENT LESS RADICAL SURGERIES THAN I HAD.

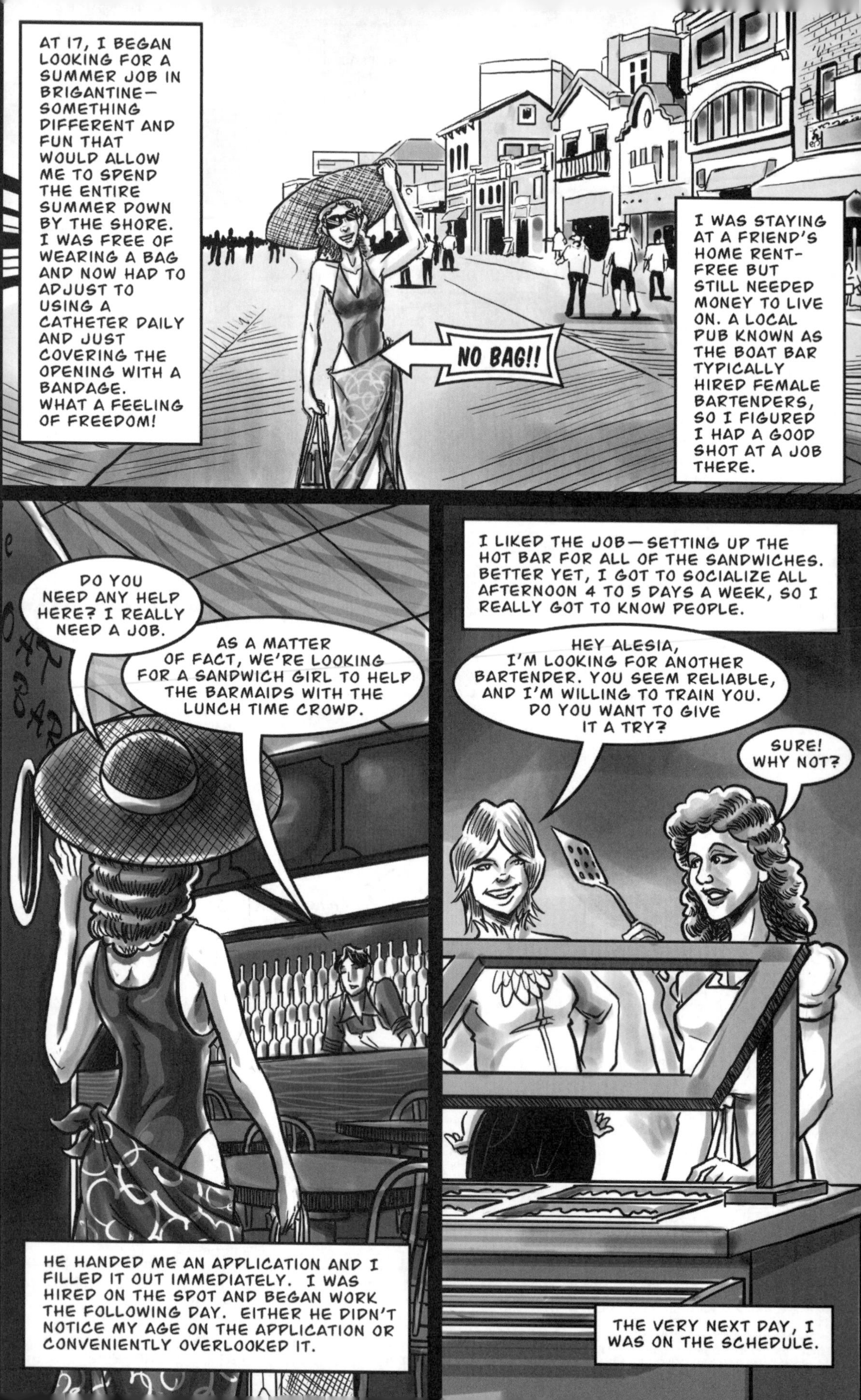
AT 17, I BEGAN LOOKING FOR A SUMMER JOB IN BRIGANTINE— SOMETHING DIFFERENT AND FUN THAT WOULD ALLOW ME TO SPEND THE ENTIRE SUMMER DOWN BY THE SHORE. I WAS FREE OF WEARING A BAG AND NOW HAD TO ADJUST TO USING A CATHETER DAILY AND JUST COVERING THE OPENING WITH A BANDAGE. WHAT A FEELING OF FREEDOM!
NO BAG!!
I WAS STAYING AT A FRIEND'S HOME RENT-FREE BUT STILL NEEDED MONEY TO LIVE ON. A LOCAL PUB KNOWN AS THE BOAT BAR TYPICALLY HIRED FEMALE BARTENDERS, SO I FIGURED I HAD A GOOD SHOT AT A JOB THERE.
DO YOU NEED ANY HELP HERE? I REALLY NEED A JOB.
AS A MATTER OF FACT, WE'RE LOOKING FOR A SANDWICH GIRL TO HELP THE BARMAIDS WITH THE LUNCH TIME CROWD.
HE HANDED ME AN APPLICATION AND I FILLED IT OUT IMMEDIATELY. I WAS HIRED ON THE SPOT AND BEGAN WORK THE FOLLOWING DAY. EITHER HE DIDN'T NOTICE MY AGE ON THE APPLICATION OR CONVENIENTLY OVERLOOKED IT.
I LIKED THE JOB—SETTING UP THE HOT BAR FOR ALL OF THE SANDWICHES. BETTER YET, I GOT TO SOCIALIZE ALL AFTERNOON 4 TO 5 DAYS A WEEK, SO I REALLY GOT TO KNOW PEOPLE.
HEY ALESIA, I'M LOOKING FOR ANOTHER BARTENDER. YOU SEEM RELIABLE, AND I'M WILLING TO TRAIN YOU. DO YOU WANT TO GIVE IT A TRY?
SURE! WHY NOT?
THE VERY NEXT DAY, I WAS ON THE SCHEDULE.

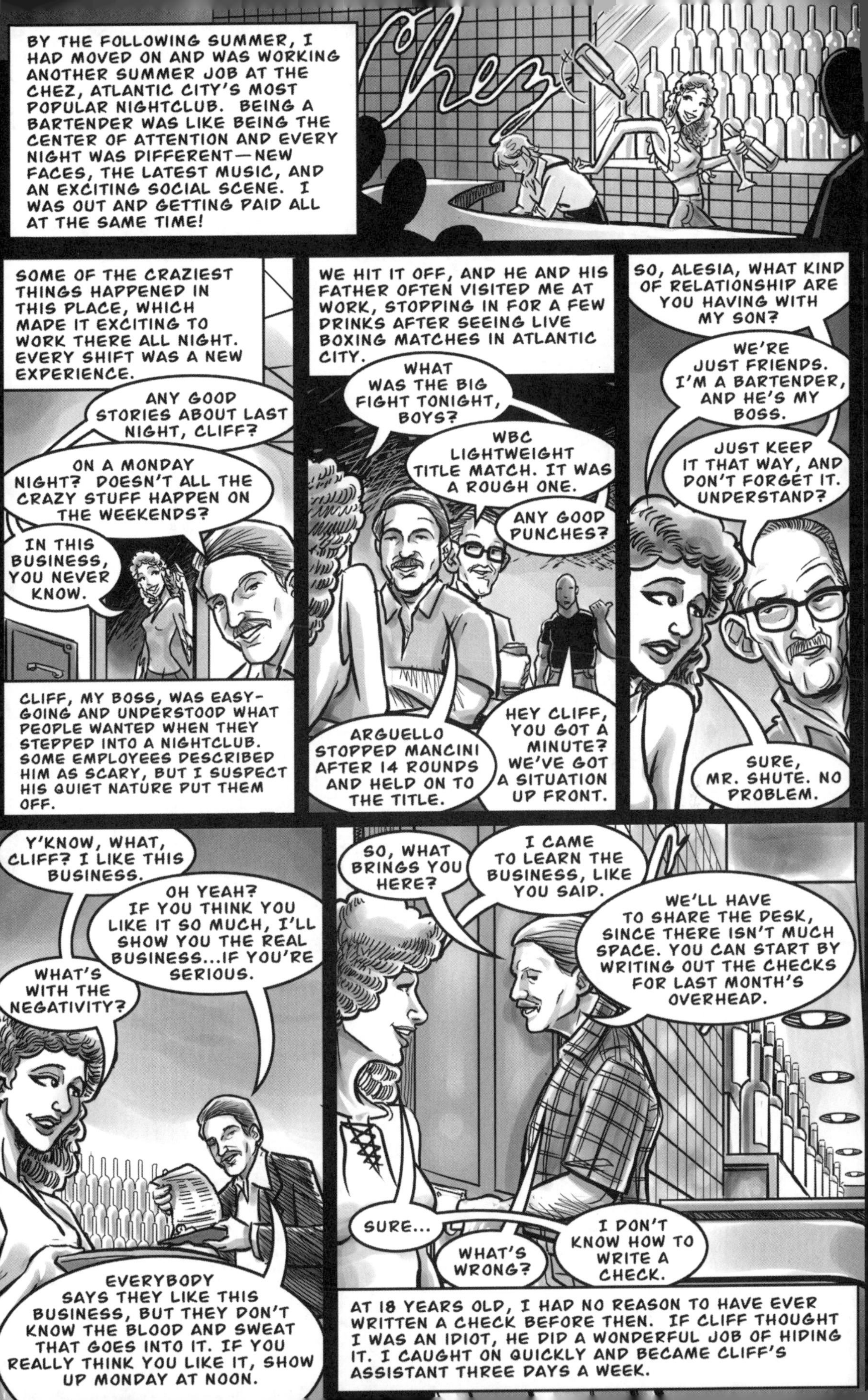
BY THE FOLLOWING SUMMER, I HAD MOVED ON AND WAS WORKING ANOTHER SUMMER JOB AT THE CHEZ, ATLANTIC CITY'S MOST POPULAR NIGHTCLUB. BEING A BARTENDER WAS LIKE BEING THE CENTER OF ATTENTION AND EVERY NIGHT WAS DIFFERENT—NEW FACES, THE LATEST MUSIC, AND AN EXCITING SOCIAL SCENE. I WAS OUT AND GETTING PAID ALL AT THE SAME TIME!
Chez
SOME OF THE CRAZIEST THINGS HAPPENED IN THIS PLACE, WHICH MADE IT EXCITING TO WORK THERE ALL NIGHT. EVERY SHIFT WAS A NEW EXPERIENCE.
ANY GOOD STORIES ABOUT LAST NIGHT, CLIFF?
ON A MONDAY NIGHT? DOESN'T ALL THE CRAZY STUFF HAPPEN ON THE WEEKENDS?
IN THIS BUSINESS, YOU NEVER KNOW.
CLIFF, MY BOSS, WAS EASY-GOING AND UNDERSTOOD WHAT PEOPLE WANTED WHEN THEY STEPPED INTO A NIGHTCLUB. SOME EMPLOYEES DESCRIBED HIM AS SCARY, BUT I SUSPECT HIS QUIET NATURE PUT THEM OFF.
WE HIT IT OFF, AND HE AND HIS FATHER OFTEN VISITED ME AT WORK, STOPPING IN FOR A FEW DRINKS AFTER SEEING LIVE BOXING MATCHES IN ATLANTIC CITY.
WHAT WAS THE BIG FIGHT TONIGHT, BOYS?
WBC LIGHTWEIGHT TITLE MATCH. IT WAS A ROUGH ONE.
ANY GOOD PUNCHES?
ARGUELLO STOPPED MANCINI AFTER 14 ROUNDS AND HELD ON TO THE TITLE.
HEY CLIFF, YOU GOT A MINUTE? WE'VE GOT A SITUATION UP FRONT.
SO, ALESIA, WHAT KIND OF RELATIONSHIP ARE YOU HAVING WITH MY SON?
WE'RE JUST FRIENDS. I'M A BARTENDER, AND HE'S MY BOSS.
JUST KEEP IT THAT WAY, AND DON'T FORGET IT. UNDERSTAND?
SURE, MR. SHUTE. NO PROBLEM.
Y'KNOW, WHAT, CLIFF? I LIKE THIS BUSINESS.
OH YEAH? IF YOU THINK YOU LIKE IT SO MUCH, I'LL SHOW YOU THE REAL BUSINESS...IF YOU'RE SERIOUS.
WHAT'S WITH THE NEGATIVITY?
EVERYBODY SAYS THEY LIKE THIS BUSINESS, BUT THEY DON'T KNOW THE BLOOD AND SWEAT THAT GOES INTO IT. IF YOU REALLY THINK YOU LIKE IT, SHOW UP MONDAY AT NOON.
SO, WHAT BRINGS YOU HERE?
I CAME TO LEARN THE BUSINESS, LIKE YOU SAID.
WE'LL HAVE TO SHARE THE DESK, SINCE THERE ISN'T MUCH SPACE. YOU CAN START BY WRITING OUT THE CHECKS FOR LAST MONTH'S OVERHEAD.
SURE...
WHAT'S WRONG?
I DON'T KNOW HOW TO WRITE A CHECK.
AT 18 YEARS OLD, I HAD NO REASON TO HAVE EVER WRITTEN A CHECK BEFORE THEN. IF CLIFF THOUGHT I WAS AN IDIOT, HE DID A WONDERFUL JOB OF HIDING IT. I CAUGHT ON QUICKLY AND BECAME CLIFF'S ASSISTANT THREE DAYS A WEEK.

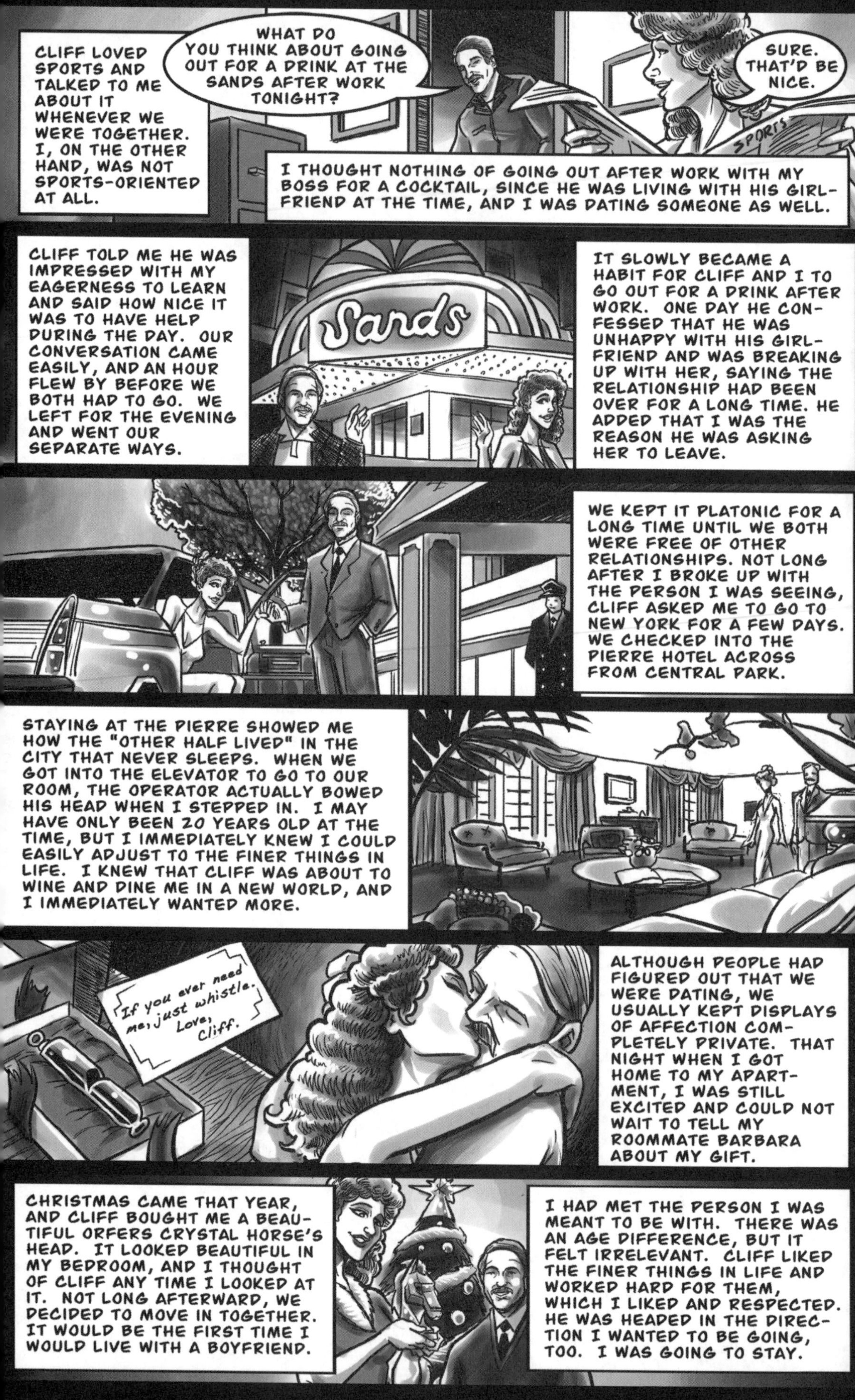

CLIFF LOVED SPORTS AND TALKED TO ME ABOUT IT WHENEVER WE WERE TOGETHER. I, ON THE OTHER HAND, WAS NOT SPORTS-ORIENTED AT ALL.
WHAT DO YOU THINK ABOUT GOING OUT FOR A DRINK AT THE SANDS AFTER WORK TONIGHT?
SURE. THAT'D BE NICE.
SPORTS
I THOUGHT NOTHING OF GOING OUT AFTER WORK WITH MY BOSS FOR A COCKTAIL, SINCE HE WAS LIVING WITH HIS GIRL-FRIEND AT THE TIME, AND I WAS DATING SOMEONE AS WELL.
CLIFF TOLD ME HE WAS IMPRESSED WITH MY EAGERNESS TO LEARN AND SAID HOW NICE IT WAS TO HAVE HELP DURING THE DAY. OUR CONVERSATION CAME EASILY, AND AN HOUR FLEW BY BEFORE WE BOTH HAD TO GO. WE LEFT FOR THE EVENING AND WENT OUR SEPARATE WAYS.
Sands
IT SLOWLY BECAME A HABIT FOR CLIFF AND I TO GO OUT FOR A DRINK AFTER WORK. ONE DAY HE CON-FESSED THAT HE WAS UNHAPPY WITH HIS GIRL-FRIEND AND WAS BREAKING UP WITH HER, SAYING THE RELATIONSHIP HAD BEEN OVER FOR A LONG TIME. HE ADDED THAT I WAS THE REASON HE WAS ASKING HER TO LEAVE.
WE KEPT IT PLATONIC FOR A LONG TIME UNTIL WE BOTH WERE FREE OF OTHER RELATIONSHIPS. NOT LONG AFTER I BROKE UP WITH THE PERSON I WAS SEEING, CLIFF ASKED ME TO GO TO NEW YORK FOR A FEW DAYS. WE CHECKED INTO THE PIERRE HOTEL ACROSS FROM CENTRAL PARK.
STAYING AT THE PIERRE SHOWED ME HOW THE "OTHER HALF LIVED" IN THE CITY THAT NEVER SLEEPS. WHEN WE GOT INTO THE ELEVATOR TO GO TO OUR ROOM, THE OPERATOR ACTUALLY BOWED HIS HEAD WHEN I STEPPED IN. I MAY HAVE ONLY BEEN 20 YEARS OLD AT THE TIME, BUT I IMMEDIATELY KNEW I COULD EASILY ADJUST TO THE FINER THINGS IN LIFE. I KNEW THAT CLIFF WAS ABOUT TO WINE AND DINE ME IN A NEW WORLD, AND I IMMEDIATELY WANTED MORE.
If you ever need me, just whistle. Love, Cliff.
ALTHOUGH PEOPLE HAD FIGURED OUT THAT WE WERE DATING, WE USUALLY KEPT DISPLAYS OF AFFECTION COM-PLETELY PRIVATE. THAT NIGHT WHEN I GOT HOME TO MY APART-MENT, I WAS STILL EXCITED AND COULD NOT WAIT TO TELL MY ROOMMATE BARBARA ABOUT MY GIFT.
CHRISTMAS CAME THAT YEAR, AND CLIFF BOUGHT ME A BEAU-TIFUL ORFERS CRYSTAL HORSE'S HEAD. IT LOOKED BEAUTIFUL IN MY BEDROOM, AND I THOUGHT OF CLIFF ANY TIME I LOOKED AT IT. NOT LONG AFTERWARD, WE DECIDED TO MOVE IN TOGETHER. IT WOULD BE THE FIRST TIME I WOULD LIVE WITH A BOYFRIEND.
I HAD MET THE PERSON I WAS MEANT TO BE WITH. THERE WAS AN AGE DIFFERENCE, BUT IT FELT IRRELEVANT. CLIFF LIKED THE FINER THINGS IN LIFE AND WORKED HARD FOR THEM, WHICH I LIKED AND RESPECTED. HE WAS HEADED IN THE DIREC-TION I WANTED TO BE GOING, TOO. I WAS GOING TO STAY.

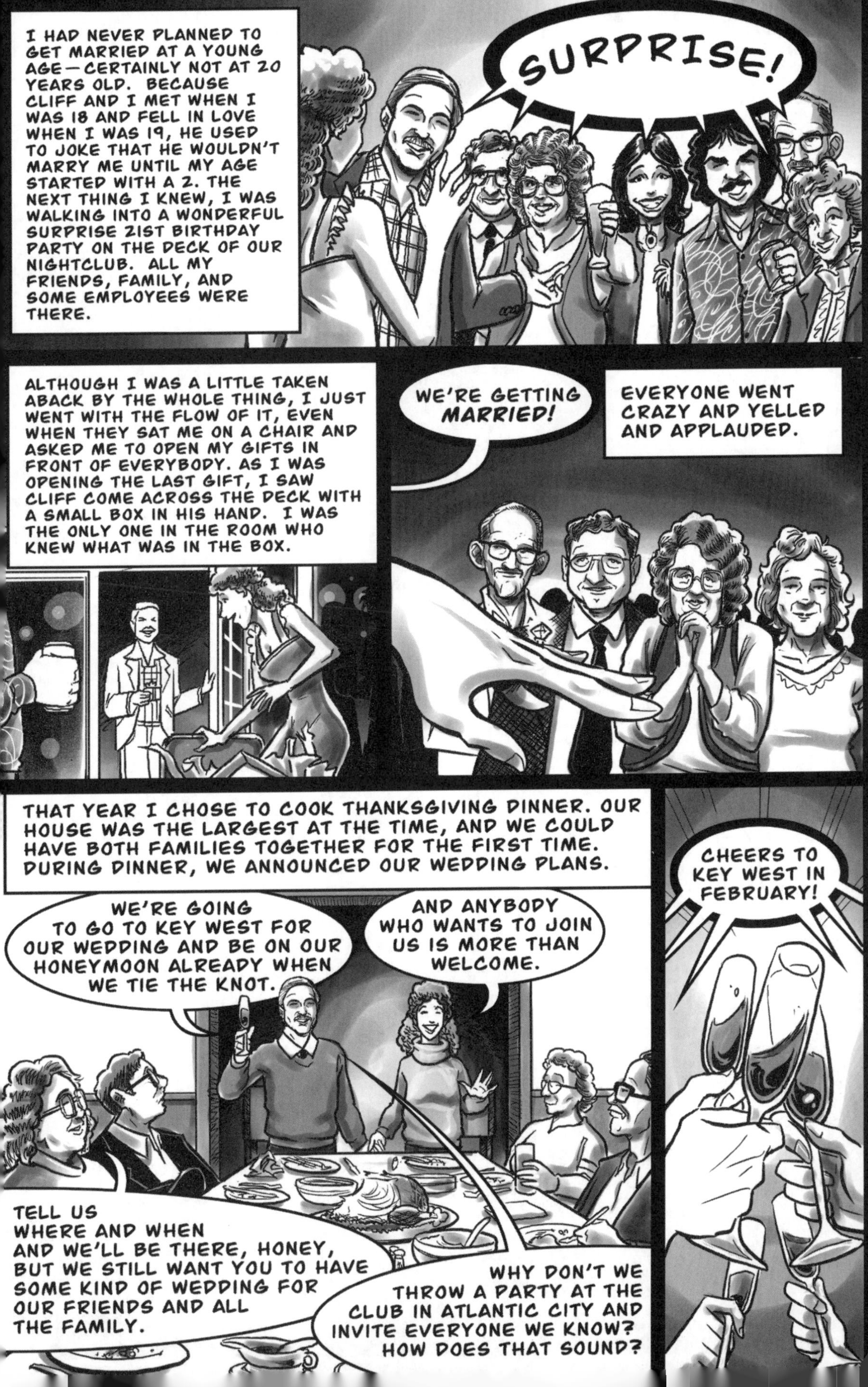
I HAD NEVER PLANNED TO GET MARRIED AT A YOUNG AGE—CERTAINLY NOT AT 20 YEARS OLD. BECAUSE CLIFF AND I MET WHEN I WAS 18 AND FELL IN LOVE WHEN I WAS 19, HE USED TO JOKE THAT HE WOULDN'T MARRY ME UNTIL MY AGE STARTED WITH A 2. THE NEXT THING I KNEW, I WAS WALKING INTO A WONDERFUL SURPRISE 21ST BIRTHDAY PARTY ON THE DECK OF OUR NIGHTCLUB. ALL MY FRIENDS, FAMILY, AND SOME EMPLOYEES WERE THERE.
SURPRISE!
ALTHOUGH I WAS A LITTLE TAKEN ABACK BY THE WHOLE THING, I JUST WENT WITH THE FLOW OF IT, EVEN WHEN THEY SAT ME ON A CHAIR AND ASKED ME TO OPEN MY GIFTS IN FRONT OF EVERYBODY. AS I WAS OPENING THE LAST GIFT, I SAW CLIFF COME ACROSS THE DECK WITH A SMALL BOX IN HIS HAND. I WAS THE ONLY ONE IN THE ROOM WHO KNEW WHAT WAS IN THE BOX.
WE'RE GETTING *MARRIED!*
EVERYONE WENT CRAZY AND YELLED AND APPLAUDED.
THAT YEAR I CHOSE TO COOK THANKSGIVING DINNER. OUR HOUSE WAS THE LARGEST AT THE TIME, AND WE COULD HAVE BOTH FAMILIES TOGETHER FOR THE FIRST TIME. DURING DINNER, WE ANNOUNCED OUR WEDDING PLANS.
WE'RE GOING TO GO TO KEY WEST FOR OUR WEDDING AND BE ON OUR HONEYMOON ALREADY WHEN WE TIE THE KNOT.
AND ANYBODY WHO WANTS TO JOIN US IS MORE THAN WELCOME.
TELL US WHERE AND WHEN AND WE'LL BE THERE, HONEY, BUT WE STILL WANT YOU TO HAVE SOME KIND OF WEDDING FOR OUR FRIENDS AND ALL THE FAMILY.
WHY DON'T WE THROW A PARTY AT THE CLUB IN ATLANTIC CITY AND INVITE EVERYONE WE KNOW? HOW DOES THAT SOUND?
CHEERS TO KEY WEST IN FEBRUARY!

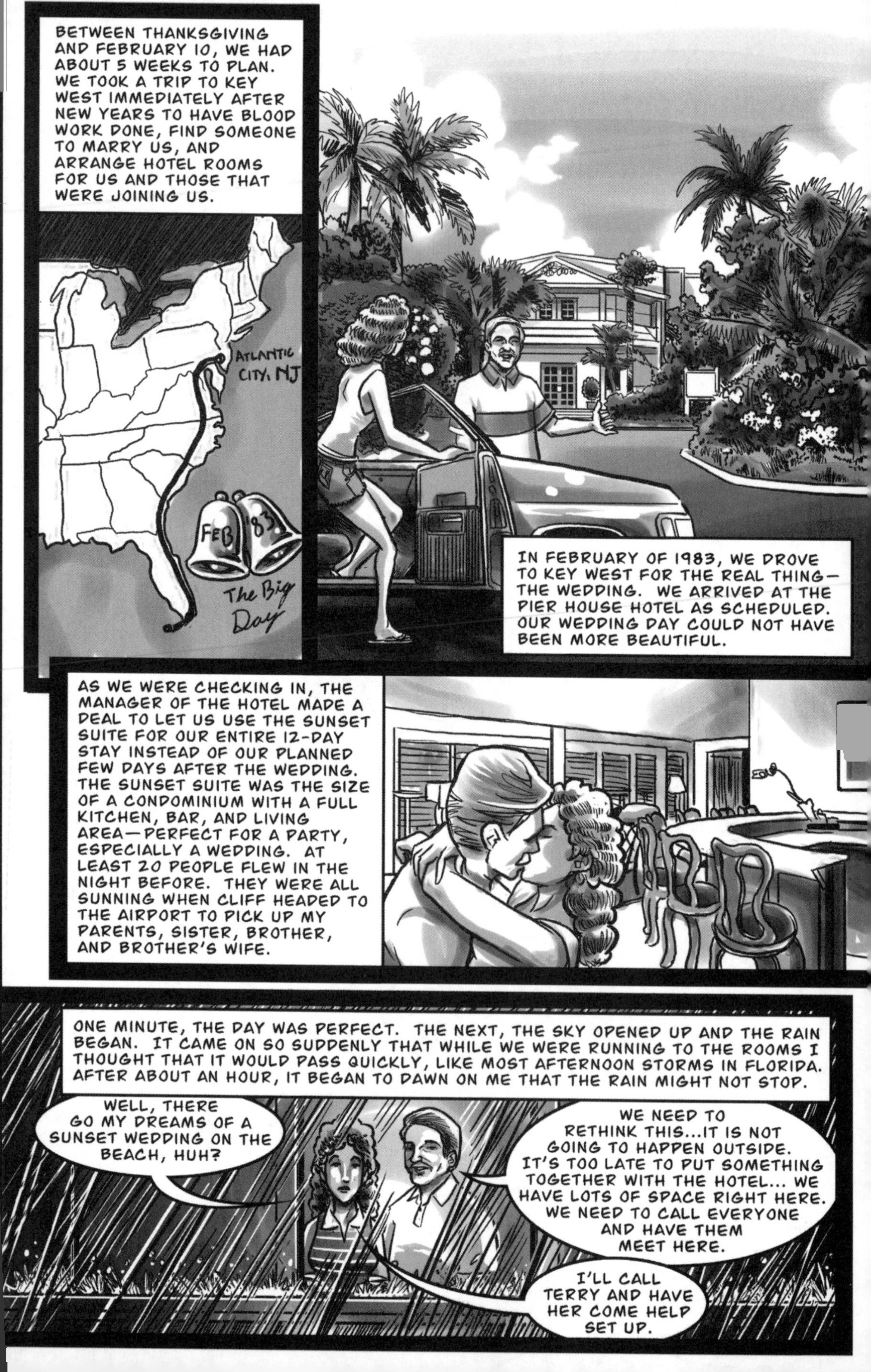
BETWEEN THANKSGIVING AND FEBRUARY 10, WE HAD ABOUT 5 WEEKS TO PLAN. WE TOOK A TRIP TO KEY WEST IMMEDIATELY AFTER NEW YEARS TO HAVE BLOOD WORK DONE, FIND SOMEONE TO MARRY US, AND ARRANGE HOTEL ROOMS FOR US AND THOSE THAT WERE JOINING US.
ATLANTIC CITY, NJ
FEB '83
The Big Day
IN FEBRUARY OF 1983, WE DROVE TO KEY WEST FOR THE REAL THING—THE WEDDING. WE ARRIVED AT THE PIER HOUSE HOTEL AS SCHEDULED. OUR WEDDING DAY COULD NOT HAVE BEEN MORE BEAUTIFUL.
AS WE WERE CHECKING IN, THE MANAGER OF THE HOTEL MADE A DEAL TO LET US USE THE SUNSET SUITE FOR OUR ENTIRE 12-DAY STAY INSTEAD OF OUR PLANNED FEW DAYS AFTER THE WEDDING. THE SUNSET SUITE WAS THE SIZE OF A CONDOMINIUM WITH A FULL KITCHEN, BAR, AND LIVING AREA—PERFECT FOR A PARTY, ESPECIALLY A WEDDING. AT LEAST 20 PEOPLE FLEW IN THE NIGHT BEFORE. THEY WERE ALL SUNNING WHEN CLIFF HEADED TO THE AIRPORT TO PICK UP MY PARENTS, SISTER, BROTHER, AND BROTHER'S WIFE.
ONE MINUTE, THE DAY WAS PERFECT. THE NEXT, THE SKY OPENED UP AND THE RAIN BEGAN. IT CAME ON SO SUDDENLY THAT WHILE WE WERE RUNNING TO THE ROOMS I THOUGHT THAT IT WOULD PASS QUICKLY, LIKE MOST AFTERNOON STORMS IN FLORIDA. AFTER ABOUT AN HOUR, IT BEGAN TO DAWN ON ME THAT THE RAIN MIGHT NOT STOP.
WELL, THERE GO MY DREAMS OF A SUNSET WEDDING ON THE BEACH, HUH?
WE NEED TO RETHINK THIS...IT IS NOT GOING TO HAPPEN OUTSIDE. IT'S TOO LATE TO PUT SOMETHING TOGETHER WITH THE HOTEL... WE HAVE LOTS OF SPACE RIGHT HERE. WE NEED TO CALL EVERYONE AND HAVE THEM MEET HERE.
I'LL CALL TERRY AND HAVE HER COME HELP SET UP.

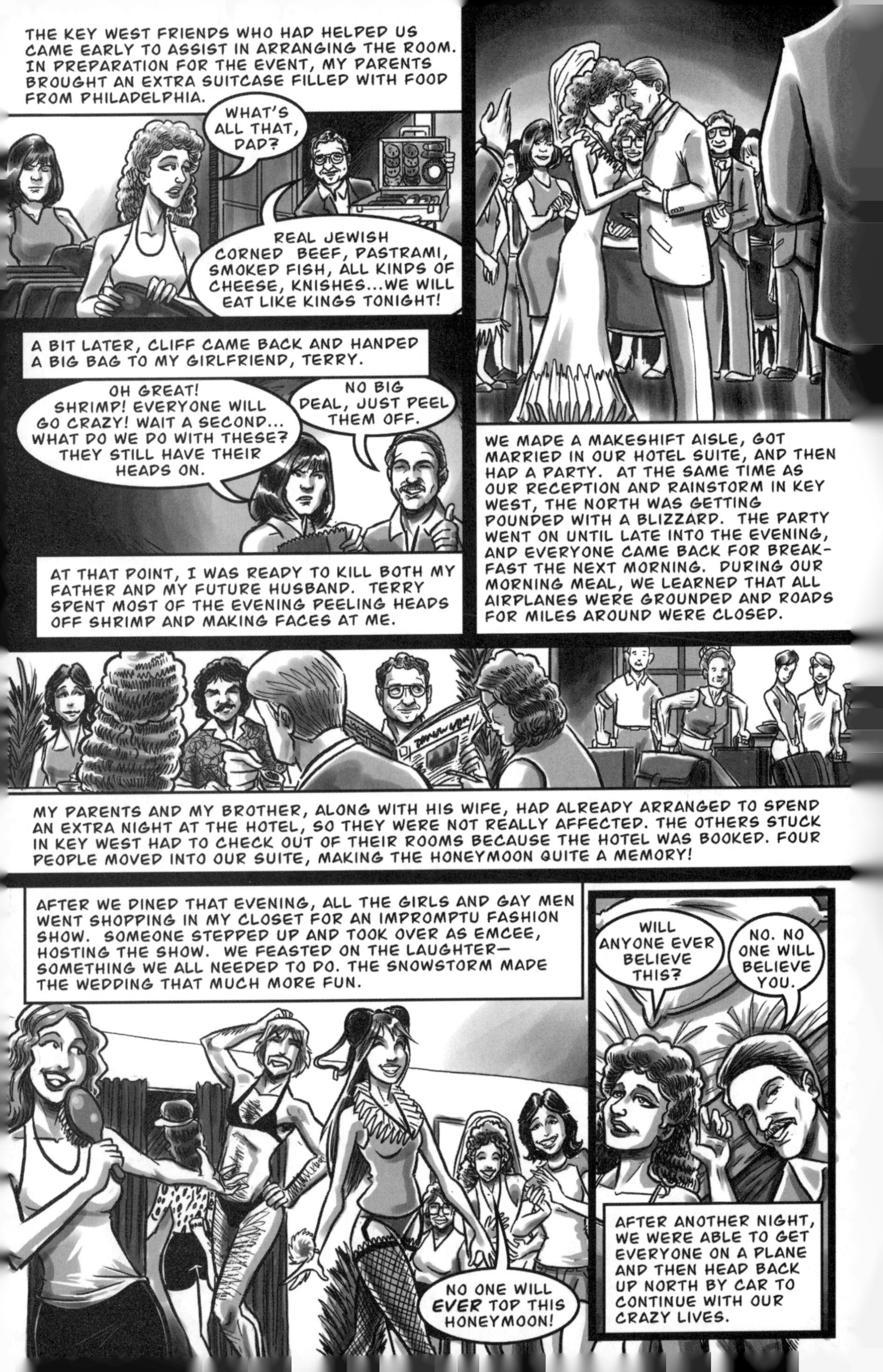
THE KEY WEST FRIENDS WHO HAD HELPED US CAME EARLY TO ASSIST IN ARRANGING THE ROOM. IN PREPARATION FOR THE EVENT, MY PARENTS BROUGHT AN EXTRA SUITCASE FILLED WITH FOOD FROM PHILADELPHIA.
WHAT'S ALL THAT, DAD?
REAL JEWISH CORNED BEEF, PASTRAMI, SMOKED FISH, ALL KINDS OF CHEESE, KNISHES...WE WILL EAT LIKE KINGS TONIGHT!
A BIT LATER, CLIFF CAME BACK AND HANDED A BIG BAG TO MY GIRLFRIEND, TERRY.
OH GREAT! SHRIMP! EVERYONE WILL GO CRAZY! WAIT A SECOND... WHAT DO WE DO WITH THESE? THEY STILL HAVE THEIR HEADS ON.
NO BIG DEAL, JUST PEEL THEM OFF.
AT THAT POINT, I WAS READY TO KILL BOTH MY FATHER AND MY FUTURE HUSBAND. TERRY SPENT MOST OF THE EVENING PEELING HEADS OFF SHRIMP AND MAKING FACES AT ME.
WE MADE A MAKESHIFT AISLE, GOT MARRIED IN OUR HOTEL SUITE, AND THEN HAD A PARTY. AT THE SAME TIME AS OUR RECEPTION AND RAINSTORM IN KEY WEST, THE NORTH WAS GETTING POUNDED WITH A BLIZZARD. THE PARTY WENT ON UNTIL LATE INTO THE EVENING, AND EVERYONE CAME BACK FOR BREAKFAST THE NEXT MORNING. DURING OUR MORNING MEAL, WE LEARNED THAT ALL AIRPLANES WERE GROUNDED AND ROADS FOR MILES AROUND WERE CLOSED.
MY PARENTS AND MY BROTHER, ALONG WITH HIS WIFE, HAD ALREADY ARRANGED TO SPEND AN EXTRA NIGHT AT THE HOTEL, SO THEY WERE NOT REALLY AFFECTED. THE OTHERS STUCK IN KEY WEST HAD TO CHECK OUT OF THEIR ROOMS BECAUSE THE HOTEL WAS BOOKED. FOUR PEOPLE MOVED INTO OUR SUITE, MAKING THE HONEYMOON QUITE A MEMORY!
AFTER WE DINED THAT EVENING, ALL THE GIRLS AND GAY MEN WENT SHOPPING IN MY CLOSET FOR AN IMPROMPTU FASHION SHOW. SOMEONE STEPPED UP AND TOOK OVER AS EMCEE, HOSTING THE SHOW. WE FEASTED ON THE LAUGHTER—SOMETHING WE ALL NEEDED TO DO. THE SNOWSTORM MADE THE WEDDING THAT MUCH MORE FUN.
NO ONE WILL EVER TOP THIS HONEYMOON!
WILL ANYONE EVER BELIEVE THIS?
NO. NO ONE WILL BELIEVE YOU.
AFTER ANOTHER NIGHT, WE WERE ABLE TO GET EVERYONE ON A PLANE AND THEN HEAD BACK UP NORTH BY CAR TO CONTINUE WITH OUR CRAZY LIVES.

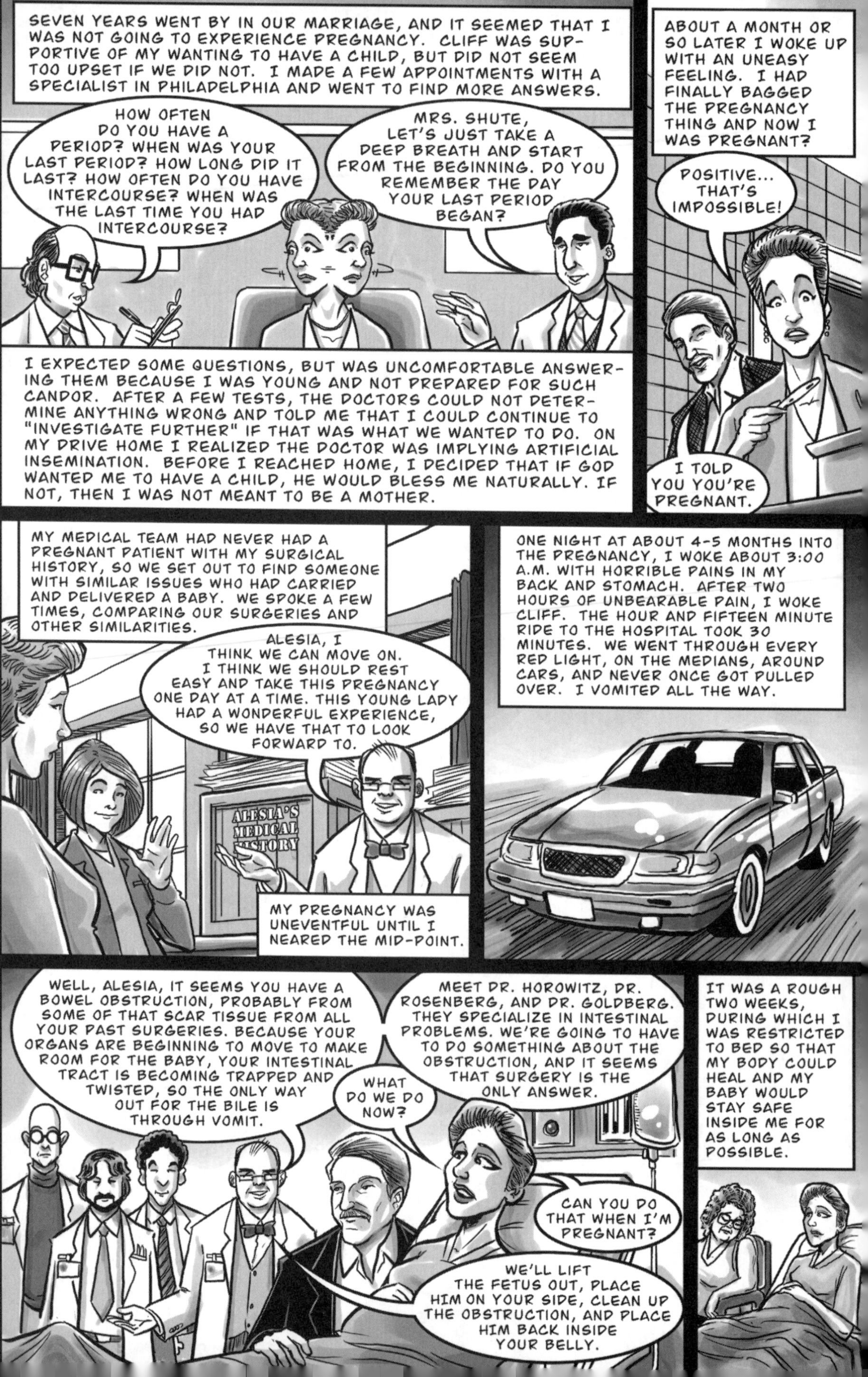
SEVEN YEARS WENT BY IN OUR MARRIAGE, AND IT SEEMED THAT I WAS NOT GOING TO EXPERIENCE PREGNANCY. CLIFF WAS SUPPORTIVE OF MY WANTING TO HAVE A CHILD, BUT DID NOT SEEM TOO UPSET IF WE DID NOT. I MADE A FEW APPOINTMENTS WITH A SPECIALIST IN PHILADELPHIA AND WENT TO FIND MORE ANSWERS.
HOW OFTEN DO YOU HAVE A PERIOD? WHEN WAS YOUR LAST PERIOD? HOW LONG DID IT LAST? HOW OFTEN DO YOU HAVE INTERCOURSE? WHEN WAS THE LAST TIME YOU HAD INTERCOURSE?
MRS. SHUTE, LET'S JUST TAKE A DEEP BREATH AND START FROM THE BEGINNING. DO YOU REMEMBER THE DAY YOUR LAST PERIOD BEGAN?
I EXPECTED SOME QUESTIONS, BUT WAS UNCOMFORTABLE ANSWERING THEM BECAUSE I WAS YOUNG AND NOT PREPARED FOR SUCH CANDOR. AFTER A FEW TESTS, THE DOCTORS COULD NOT DETERMINE ANYTHING WRONG AND TOLD ME THAT I COULD CONTINUE TO "INVESTIGATE FURTHER" IF THAT WAS WHAT WE WANTED TO DO. ON MY DRIVE HOME I REALIZED THE DOCTOR WAS IMPLYING ARTIFICIAL INSEMINATION. BEFORE I REACHED HOME, I DECIDED THAT IF GOD WANTED ME TO HAVE A CHILD, HE WOULD BLESS ME NATURALLY. IF NOT, THEN I WAS NOT MEANT TO BE A MOTHER.
ABOUT A MONTH OR SO LATER I WOKE UP WITH AN UNEASY FEELING. I HAD FINALLY BAGGED THE PREGNANCY THING AND NOW I WAS PREGNANT?
POSITIVE... THAT'S IMPOSSIBLE!
I TOLD YOU YOU'RE PREGNANT.
MY MEDICAL TEAM HAD NEVER HAD A PREGNANT PATIENT WITH MY SURGICAL HISTORY, SO WE SET OUT TO FIND SOMEONE WITH SIMILAR ISSUES WHO HAD CARRIED AND DELIVERED A BABY. WE SPOKE A FEW TIMES, COMPARING OUR SURGERIES AND OTHER SIMILARITIES.
ALESIA, I THINK WE CAN MOVE ON. I THINK WE SHOULD REST EASY AND TAKE THIS PREGNANCY ONE DAY AT A TIME. THIS YOUNG LADY HAD A WONDERFUL EXPERIENCE, SO WE HAVE THAT TO LOOK FORWARD TO.
ALESIA'S MEDICAL
MY PREGNANCY WAS UNEVENTFUL UNTIL I NEARED THE MID-POINT.
ONE NIGHT AT ABOUT 4-5 MONTHS INTO THE PREGNANCY, I WOKE ABOUT 3:00 A.M. WITH HORRIBLE PAINS IN MY BACK AND STOMACH. AFTER TWO HOURS OF UNBEARABLE PAIN, I WOKE CLIFF. THE HOUR AND FIFTEEN MINUTE RIDE TO THE HOSPITAL TOOK 30 MINUTES. WE WENT THROUGH EVERY RED LIGHT, ON THE MEDIANS, AROUND CARS, AND NEVER ONCE GOT PULLED OVER. I VOMITED ALL THE WAY.
WELL, ALESIA, IT SEEMS YOU HAVE A BOWEL OBSTRUCTION, PROBABLY FROM SOME OF THAT SCAR TISSUE FROM ALL YOUR PAST SURGERIES. BECAUSE YOUR ORGANS ARE BEGINNING TO MOVE TO MAKE ROOM FOR THE BABY, YOUR INTESTINAL TRACT IS BECOMING TRAPPED AND TWISTED, SO THE ONLY WAY OUT FOR THE BILE IS THROUGH VOMIT.
WHAT DO WE DO NOW?
MEET DR. HOROWITZ, DR. ROSENBERG, AND DR. GOLDBERG. THEY SPECIALIZE IN INTESTINAL PROBLEMS. WE'RE GOING TO HAVE TO DO SOMETHING ABOUT THE OBSTRUCTION, AND IT SEEMS THAT SURGERY IS THE ONLY ANSWER.
CAN YOU DO THAT WHEN I'M PREGNANT?
WE'LL LIFT THE FETUS OUT, PLACE HIM ON YOUR SIDE, CLEAN UP THE OBSTRUCTION, AND PLACE HIM BACK INSIDE YOUR BELLY.
IT WAS A ROUGH TWO WEEKS, DURING WHICH I WAS RESTRICTED TO BED SO THAT MY BODY COULD HEAL AND MY BABY WOULD STAY SAFE INSIDE ME FOR AS LONG AS POSSIBLE.

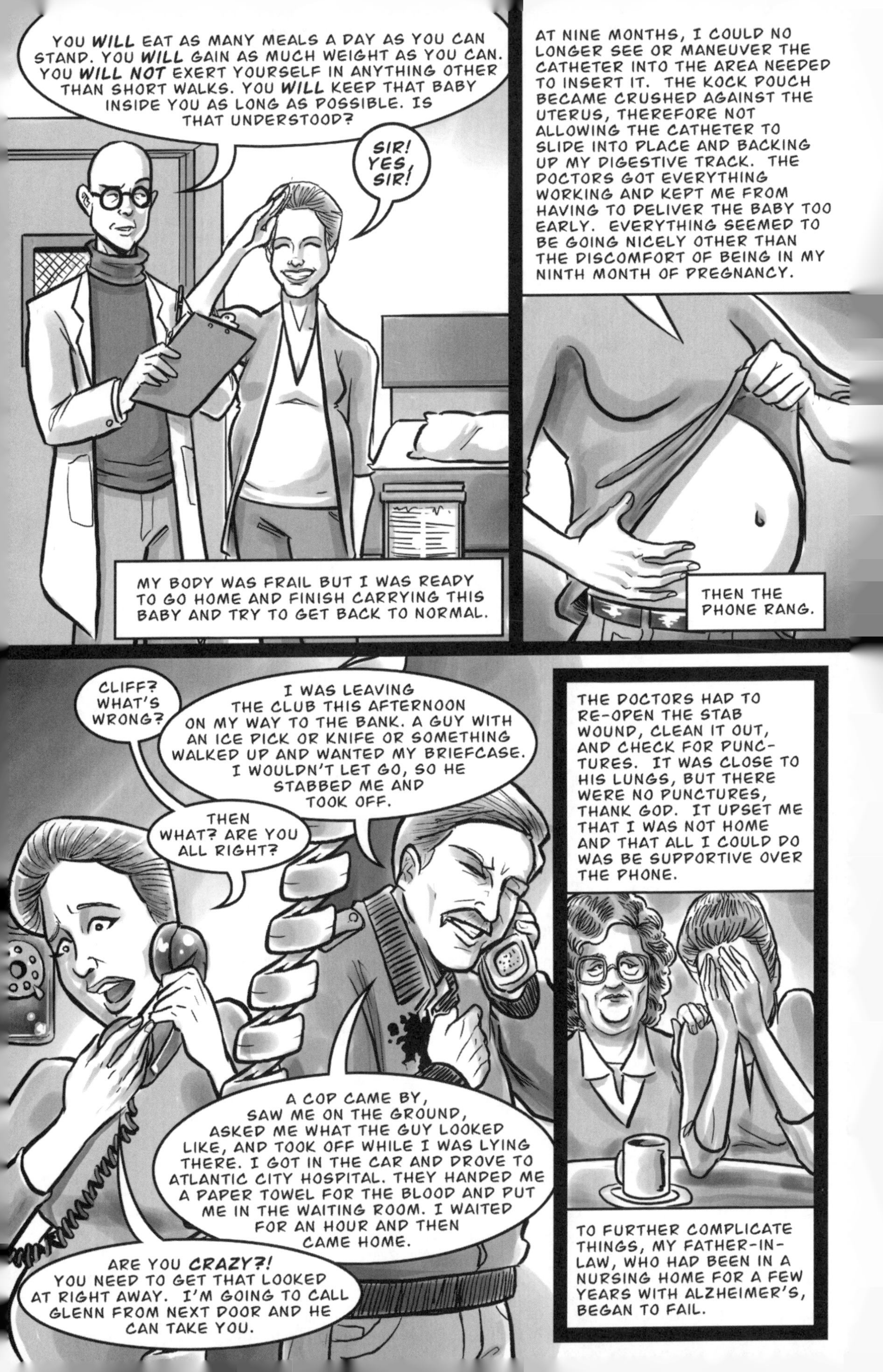
YOU WILL EAT AS MANY MEALS A DAY AS YOU CAN STAND. YOU WILL GAIN AS MUCH WEIGHT AS YOU CAN. YOU WILL NOT EXERT YOURSELF IN ANYTHING OTHER THAN SHORT WALKS. YOU WILL KEEP THAT BABY INSIDE YOU AS LONG AS POSSIBLE. IS THAT UNDERSTOOD?
SIR! YES, SIR!
MY BODY WAS FRAIL BUT I WAS READY TO GO HOME AND FINISH CARRYING THIS BABY AND TRY TO GET BACK TO NORMAL.
AT NINE MONTHS, I COULD NO LONGER SEE OR MANEUVER THE CATHETER INTO THE AREA NEEDED TO INSERT IT. THE KOCK POUCH BECAME CRUSHED AGAINST THE UTERUS, THEREFORE NOT ALLOWING THE CATHETER TO SLIDE INTO PLACE AND BACKING UP MY DIGESTIVE TRACK. THE DOCTORS GOT EVERYTHING WORKING AND KEPT ME FROM HAVING TO DELIVER THE BABY TOO EARLY. EVERYTHING SEEMED TO BE GOING NICELY OTHER THAN THE DISCOMFORT OF BEING IN MY NINTH MONTH OF PREGNANCY.
THEN THE PHONE RANG.
CLIFF? WHAT'S WRONG?
I WAS LEAVING THE CLUB THIS AFTERNOON ON MY WAY TO THE BANK. A GUY WITH AN ICE PICK OR KNIFE OR SOMETHING WALKED UP AND WANTED MY BRIEFCASE. I WOULDN'T LET GO, SO HE STABBED ME AND TOOK OFF.
THEN WHAT? ARE YOU ALL RIGHT?
A COP CAME BY, SAW ME ON THE GROUND, ASKED ME WHAT THE GUY LOOKED LIKE, AND TOOK OFF WHILE I WAS LYING THERE. I GOT IN THE CAR AND DROVE TO ATLANTIC CITY HOSPITAL. THEY HANDED ME A PAPER TOWEL FOR THE BLOOD AND PUT ME IN THE WAITING ROOM. I WAITED FOR AN HOUR AND THEN CAME HOME.
ARE YOU CRAZY?! YOU NEED TO GET THAT LOOKED AT RIGHT AWAY. I'M GOING TO CALL GLENN FROM NEXT DOOR AND HE CAN TAKE YOU.
THE DOCTORS HAD TO RE-OPEN THE STAB WOUND, CLEAN IT OUT, AND CHECK FOR PUNCTURES. IT WAS CLOSE TO HIS LUNGS, BUT THERE WERE NO PUNCTURES, THANK GOD. IT UPSET ME THAT I WAS NOT HOME AND THAT ALL I COULD DO WAS BE SUPPORTIVE OVER THE PHONE.
TO FURTHER COMPLICATE THINGS, MY FATHER-IN-LAW, WHO HAD BEEN IN A NURSING HOME FOR A FEW YEARS WITH ALZHEIMER'S, BEGAN TO FAIL.

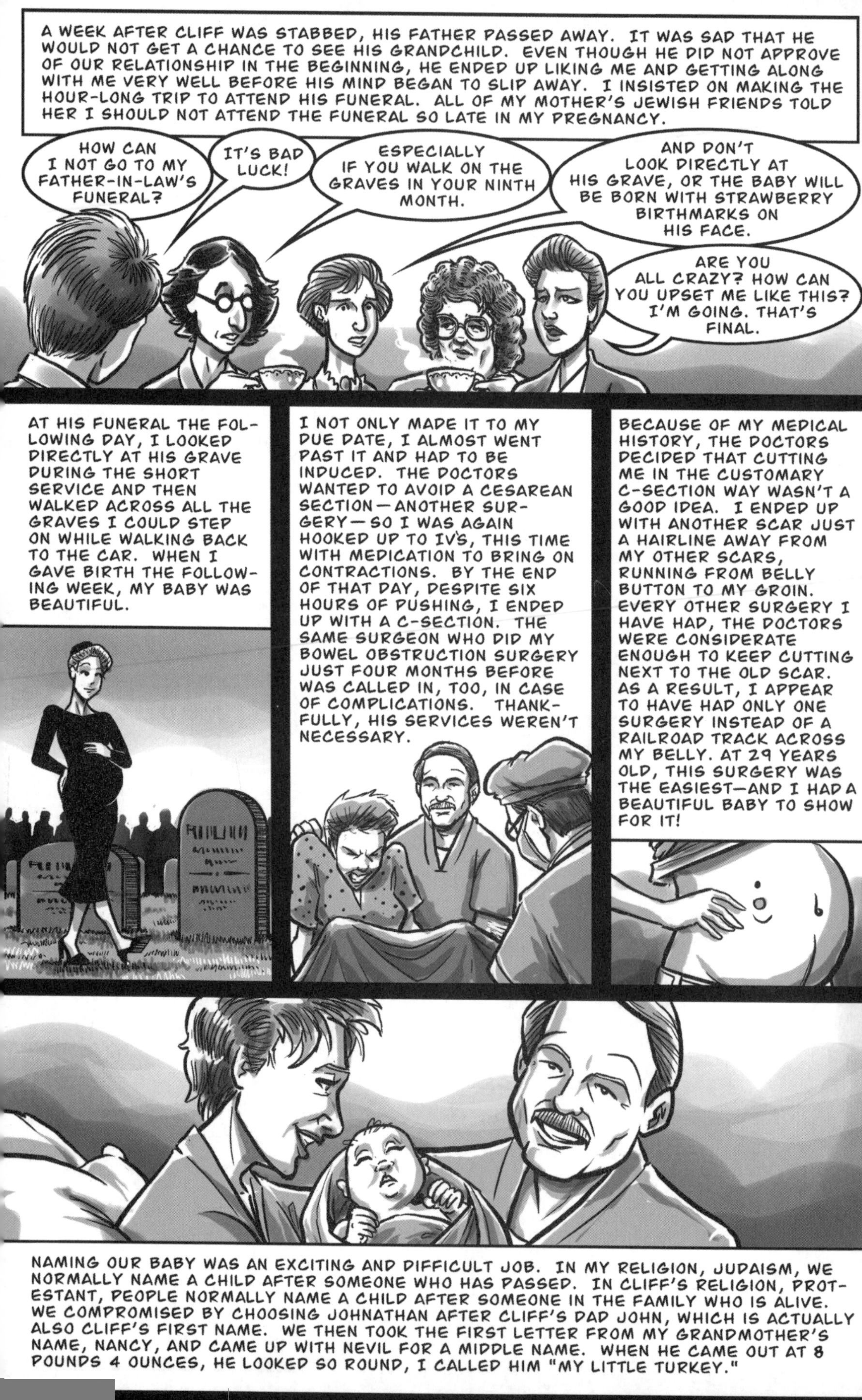
A WEEK AFTER CLIFF WAS STABBED, HIS FATHER PASSED AWAY. IT WAS SAD THAT HE WOULD NOT GET A CHANCE TO SEE HIS GRANDCHILD. EVEN THOUGH HE DID NOT APPROVE OF OUR RELATIONSHIP IN THE BEGINNING, HE ENDED UP LIKING ME AND GETTING ALONG WITH ME VERY WELL BEFORE HIS MIND BEGAN TO SLIP AWAY. I INSISTED ON MAKING THE HOUR-LONG TRIP TO ATTEND HIS FUNERAL. ALL OF MY MOTHER'S JEWISH FRIENDS TOLD HER I SHOULD NOT ATTEND THE FUNERAL SO LATE IN MY PREGNANCY.
HOW CAN I NOT GO TO MY FATHER-IN-LAW'S FUNERAL?
IT'S BAD LUCK!
ESPECIALLY IF YOU WALK ON THE GRAVES IN YOUR NINTH MONTH.
AND DON'T LOOK DIRECTLY AT HIS GRAVE, OR THE BABY WILL BE BORN WITH STRAWBERRY BIRTHMARKS ON HIS FACE.
ARE YOU ALL CRAZY? HOW CAN YOU UPSET ME LIKE THIS? I'M GOING. THAT'S FINAL.
AT HIS FUNERAL THE FOLLOWING DAY, I LOOKED DIRECTLY AT HIS GRAVE DURING THE SHORT SERVICE AND THEN WALKED ACROSS ALL THE GRAVES I COULD STEP ON WHILE WALKING BACK TO THE CAR. WHEN I GAVE BIRTH THE FOLLOWING WEEK, MY BABY WAS BEAUTIFUL.
I NOT ONLY MADE IT TO MY DUE DATE, I ALMOST WENT PAST IT AND HAD TO BE INDUCED. THE DOCTORS WANTED TO AVOID A CESAREAN SECTION—ANOTHER SURGERY—SO I WAS AGAIN HOOKED UP TO IV'S, THIS TIME WITH MEDICATION TO BRING ON CONTRACTIONS. BY THE END OF THAT DAY, DESPITE SIX HOURS OF PUSHING, I ENDED UP WITH A C-SECTION. THE SAME SURGEON WHO DID MY BOWEL OBSTRUCTION SURGERY JUST FOUR MONTHS BEFORE WAS CALLED IN, TOO, IN CASE OF COMPLICATIONS. THANKFULLY, HIS SERVICES WEREN'T NECESSARY.
BECAUSE OF MY MEDICAL HISTORY, THE DOCTORS DECIDED THAT CUTTING ME IN THE CUSTOMARY C-SECTION WAY WASN'T A GOOD IDEA. I ENDED UP WITH ANOTHER SCAR JUST A HAIRLINE AWAY FROM MY OTHER SCARS, RUNNING FROM BELLY BUTTON TO MY GROIN. EVERY OTHER SURGERY I HAVE HAD, THE DOCTORS WERE CONSIDERATE ENOUGH TO KEEP CUTTING NEXT TO THE OLD SCAR. AS A RESULT, I APPEAR TO HAVE HAD ONLY ONE SURGERY INSTEAD OF A RAILROAD TRACK ACROSS MY BELLY. AT 29 YEARS OLD, THIS SURGERY WAS THE EASIEST—AND I HAD A BEAUTIFUL BABY TO SHOW FOR IT!
NAMING OUR BABY WAS AN EXCITING AND DIFFICULT JOB. IN MY RELIGION, JUDAISM, WE NORMALLY NAME A CHILD AFTER SOMEONE WHO HAS PASSED. IN CLIFF'S RELIGION, PROTESTANT, PEOPLE NORMALLY NAME A CHILD AFTER SOMEONE IN THE FAMILY WHO IS ALIVE. WE COMPROMISED BY CHOOSING JOHNATHAN AFTER CLIFF'S DAD JOHN, WHICH IS ACTUALLY ALSO CLIFF'S FIRST NAME. WE THEN TOOK THE FIRST LETTER FROM MY GRANDMOTHER'S NAME, NANCY, AND CAME UP WITH NEVIL FOR A MIDDLE NAME. WHEN HE CAME OUT AT 8 POUNDS 4 OUNCES, HE LOOKED SO ROUND, I CALLED HIM "MY LITTLE TURKEY."

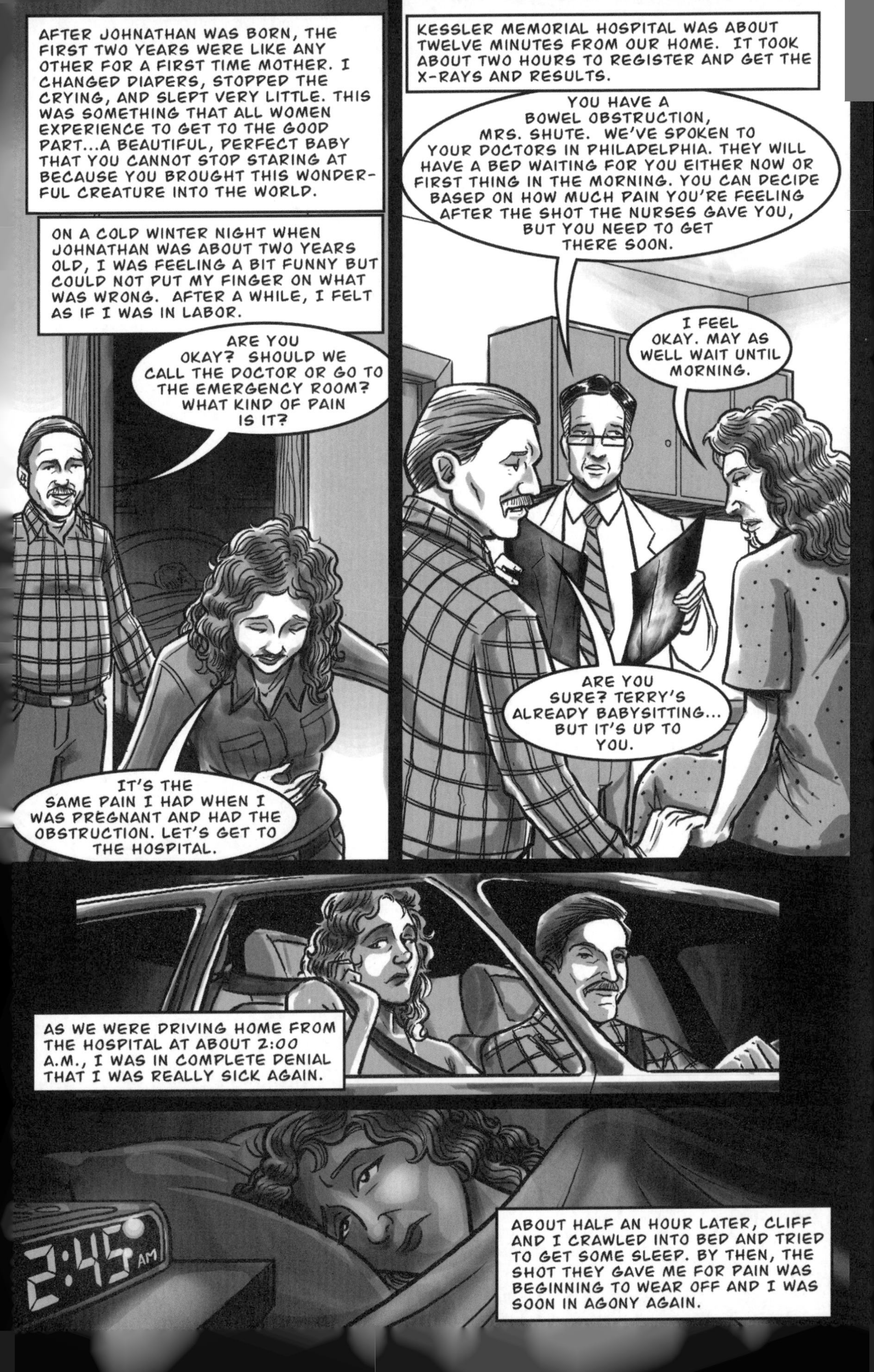
AFTER JOHNATHAN WAS BORN, THE FIRST TWO YEARS WERE LIKE ANY OTHER FOR A FIRST TIME MOTHER. I CHANGED DIAPERS, STOPPED THE CRYING, AND SLEPT VERY LITTLE. THIS WAS SOMETHING THAT ALL WOMEN EXPERIENCE TO GET TO THE GOOD PART...A BEAUTIFUL, PERFECT BABY THAT YOU CANNOT STOP STARING AT BECAUSE YOU BROUGHT THIS WONDERFUL CREATURE INTO THE WORLD.
ON A COLD WINTER NIGHT WHEN JOHNATHAN WAS ABOUT TWO YEARS OLD, I WAS FEELING A BIT FUNNY BUT COULD NOT PUT MY FINGER ON WHAT WAS WRONG. AFTER A WHILE, I FELT AS IF I WAS IN LABOR.
ARE YOU OKAY? SHOULD WE CALL THE DOCTOR OR GO TO THE EMERGENCY ROOM? WHAT KIND OF PAIN IS IT?
IT'S THE SAME PAIN I HAD WHEN I WAS PREGNANT AND HAD THE OBSTRUCTION. LET'S GET TO THE HOSPITAL.
KESSLER MEMORIAL HOSPITAL WAS ABOUT TWELVE MINUTES FROM OUR HOME. IT TOOK ABOUT TWO HOURS TO REGISTER AND GET THE X-RAYS AND RESULTS.
YOU HAVE A BOWEL OBSTRUCTION, MRS. SHUTE. WE'VE SPOKEN TO YOUR DOCTORS IN PHILADELPHIA. THEY WILL HAVE A BED WAITING FOR YOU EITHER NOW OR FIRST THING IN THE MORNING. YOU CAN DECIDE BASED ON HOW MUCH PAIN YOU'RE FEELING AFTER THE SHOT THE NURSES GAVE YOU, BUT YOU NEED TO GET THERE SOON.
I FEEL OKAY. MAY AS WELL WAIT UNTIL MORNING.
ARE YOU SURE? TERRY'S ALREADY BABYSITTING... BUT IT'S UP TO YOU.
AS WE WERE DRIVING HOME FROM THE HOSPITAL AT ABOUT 2:00 A.M., I WAS IN COMPLETE DENIAL THAT I WAS REALLY SICK AGAIN.
2:45 AM
ABOUT HALF AN HOUR LATER, CLIFF AND I CRAWLED INTO BED AND TRIED TO GET SOME SLEEP. BY THEN, THE SHOT THEY GAVE ME FOR PAIN WAS BEGINNING TO WEAR OFF AND I WAS SOON IN AGONY AGAIN.

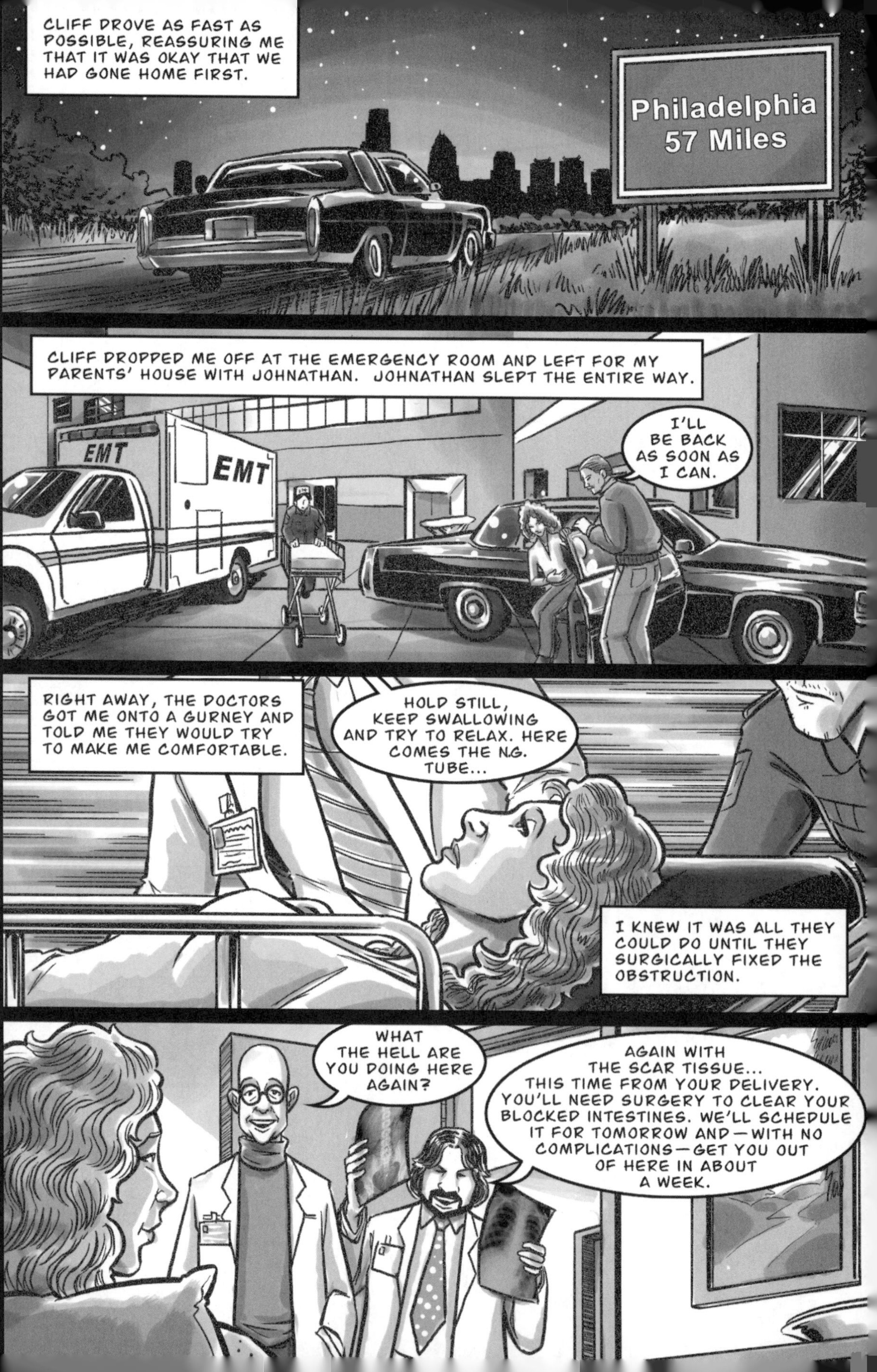
CLIFF DROVE AS FAST AS POSSIBLE, REASSURING ME THAT IT WAS OKAY THAT WE HAD GONE HOME FIRST.
Philadelphia 57 Miles
CLIFF DROPPED ME OFF AT THE EMERGENCY ROOM AND LEFT FOR MY PARENTS' HOUSE WITH JOHNATHAN. JOHNATHAN SLEPT THE ENTIRE WAY.
EMT
EMT
I'LL BE BACK AS SOON AS I CAN.
RIGHT AWAY, THE DOCTORS GOT ME ONTO A GURNEY AND TOLD ME THEY WOULD TRY TO MAKE ME COMFORTABLE.
HOLD STILL, KEEP SWALLOWING AND TRY TO RELAX. HERE COMES THE N.G. TUBE...
I KNEW IT WAS ALL THEY COULD DO UNTIL THEY SURGICALLY FIXED THE OBSTRUCTION.
WHAT THE HELL ARE YOU DOING HERE AGAIN?
AGAIN WITH THE SCAR TISSUE... THIS TIME FROM YOUR DELIVERY. YOU'LL NEED SURGERY TO CLEAR YOUR BLOCKED INTESTINES. WE'LL SCHEDULE IT FOR TOMORROW AND—WITH NO COMPLICATIONS—GET YOU OUT OF HERE IN ABOUT A WEEK.

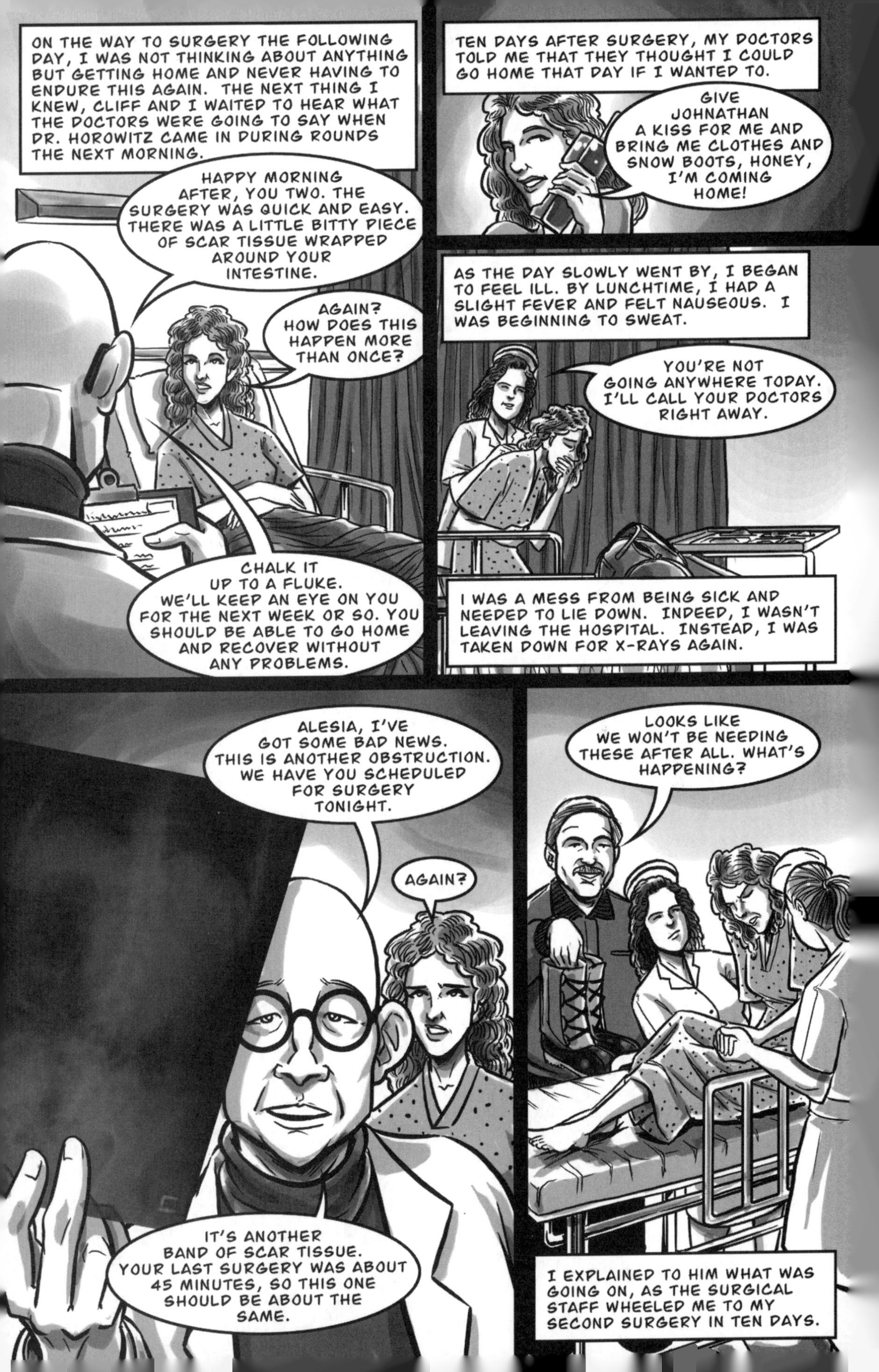
ON THE WAY TO SURGERY THE FOLLOWING DAY, I WAS NOT THINKING ABOUT ANYTHING BUT GETTING HOME AND NEVER HAVING TO ENDURE THIS AGAIN. THE NEXT THING I KNEW, CLIFF AND I WAITED TO HEAR WHAT THE DOCTORS WERE GOING TO SAY WHEN DR. HOROWITZ CAME IN DURING ROUNDS THE NEXT MORNING.
HAPPY MORNING AFTER, YOU TWO. THE SURGERY WAS QUICK AND EASY. THERE WAS A LITTLE BITTY PIECE OF SCAR TISSUE WRAPPED AROUND YOUR INTESTINE.
AGAIN? HOW DOES THIS HAPPEN MORE THAN ONCE?
CHALK IT UP TO A FLUKE. WE'LL KEEP AN EYE ON YOU FOR THE NEXT WEEK OR SO. YOU SHOULD BE ABLE TO GO HOME AND RECOVER WITHOUT ANY PROBLEMS.
TEN DAYS AFTER SURGERY, MY DOCTORS TOLD ME THAT THEY THOUGHT I COULD GO HOME THAT DAY IF I WANTED TO.
GIVE JOHNATHAN A KISS FOR ME AND BRING ME CLOTHES AND SNOW BOOTS, HONEY, I'M COMING HOME!
AS THE DAY SLOWLY WENT BY, I BEGAN TO FEEL ILL. BY LUNCHTIME, I HAD A SLIGHT FEVER AND FELT NAUSEOUS. I WAS BEGINNING TO SWEAT.
YOU'RE NOT GOING ANYWHERE TODAY. I'LL CALL YOUR DOCTORS RIGHT AWAY.
I WAS A MESS FROM BEING SICK AND NEEDED TO LIE DOWN. INDEED, I WASN'T LEAVING THE HOSPITAL. INSTEAD, I WAS TAKEN DOWN FOR X-RAYS AGAIN.
ALESIA, I'VE GOT SOME BAD NEWS. THIS IS ANOTHER OBSTRUCTION. WE HAVE YOU SCHEDULED FOR SURGERY TONIGHT.
AGAIN?
IT'S ANOTHER BAND OF SCAR TISSUE. YOUR LAST SURGERY WAS ABOUT 45 MINUTES, SO THIS ONE SHOULD BE ABOUT THE SAME.
LOOKS LIKE WE WON'T BE NEEDING THESE AFTER ALL. WHAT'S HAPPENING?
I EXPLAINED TO HIM WHAT WAS GOING ON, AS THE SURGICAL STAFF WHEELED ME TO MY SECOND SURGERY IN TEN DAYS.

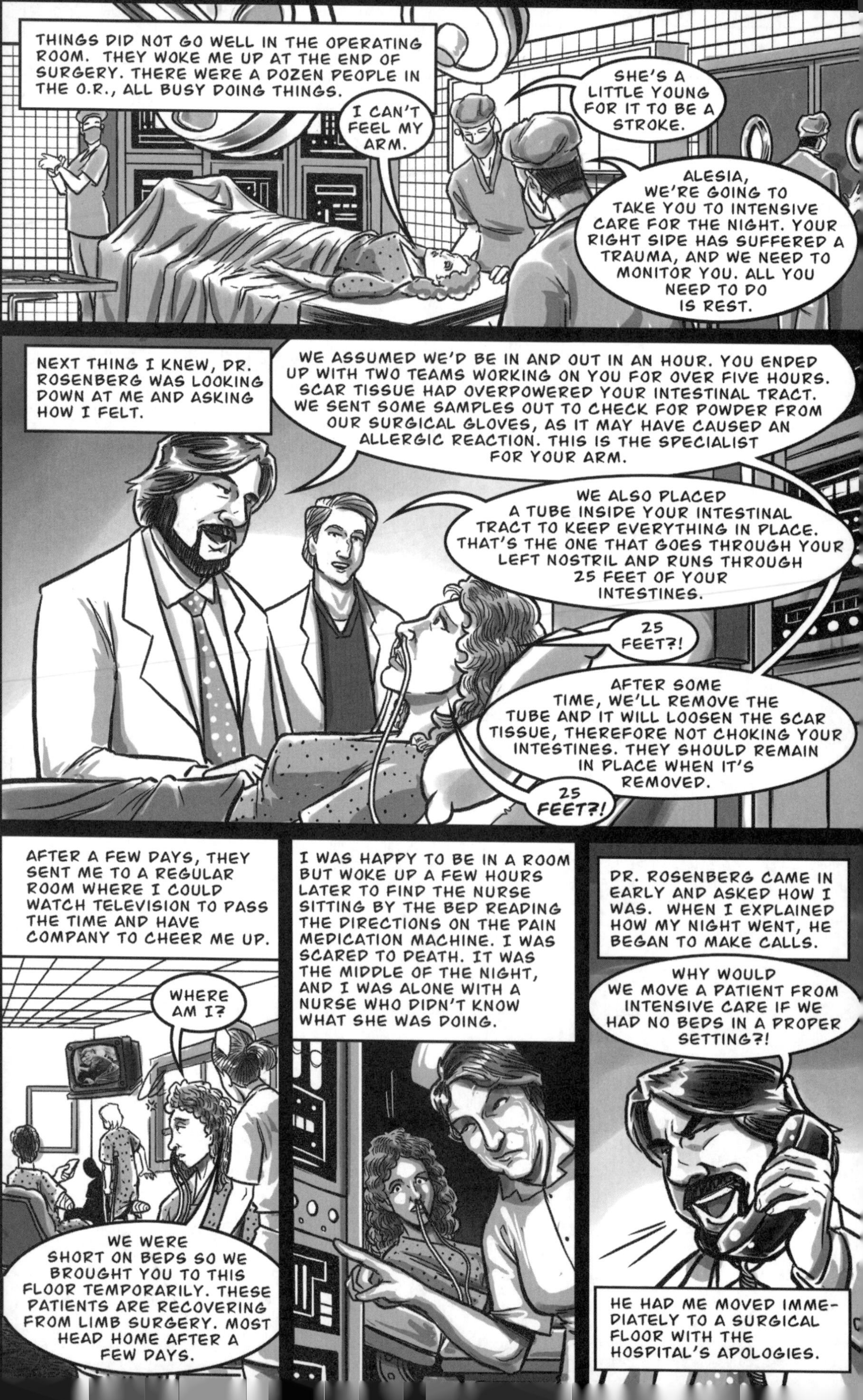
THINGS DID NOT GO WELL IN THE OPERATING ROOM. THEY WOKE ME UP AT THE END OF SURGERY. THERE WERE A DOZEN PEOPLE IN THE O.R., ALL BUSY DOING THINGS.
I CAN'T FEEL MY ARM.
SHE'S A LITTLE YOUNG FOR IT TO BE A STROKE.
ALESIA, WE'RE GOING TO TAKE YOU TO INTENSIVE CARE FOR THE NIGHT. YOUR RIGHT SIDE HAS SUFFERED A TRAUMA, AND WE NEED TO MONITOR YOU. ALL YOU NEED TO DO IS REST.
NEXT THING I KNEW, DR. ROSENBERG WAS LOOKING DOWN AT ME AND ASKING HOW I FELT.
WE ASSUMED WE'D BE IN AND OUT IN AN HOUR. YOU ENDED UP WITH TWO TEAMS WORKING ON YOU FOR OVER FIVE HOURS. SCAR TISSUE HAD OVERPOWERED YOUR INTESTINAL TRACT. WE SENT SOME SAMPLES OUT TO CHECK FOR POWDER FROM OUR SURGICAL GLOVES, AS IT MAY HAVE CAUSED AN ALLERGIC REACTION. THIS IS THE SPECIALIST FOR YOUR ARM.
WE ALSO PLACED A TUBE INSIDE YOUR INTESTINAL TRACT TO KEEP EVERYTHING IN PLACE. THAT'S THE ONE THAT GOES THROUGH YOUR LEFT NOSTRIL AND RUNS THROUGH 25 FEET OF YOUR INTESTINES.
25 FEET?!
AFTER SOME TIME, WE'LL REMOVE THE TUBE AND IT WILL LOOSEN THE SCAR TISSUE, THEREFORE NOT CHOKING YOUR INTESTINES. THEY SHOULD REMAIN IN PLACE WHEN IT'S REMOVED.
25 FEET?!
AFTER A FEW DAYS, THEY SENT ME TO A REGULAR ROOM WHERE I COULD WATCH TELEVISION TO PASS THE TIME AND HAVE COMPANY TO CHEER ME UP.
WHERE AM I?
WE WERE SHORT ON BEDS SO WE BROUGHT YOU TO THIS FLOOR TEMPORARILY. THESE PATIENTS ARE RECOVERING FROM LIMB SURGERY. MOST HEAD HOME AFTER A FEW DAYS.
I WAS HAPPY TO BE IN A ROOM BUT WOKE UP A FEW HOURS LATER TO FIND THE NURSE SITTING BY THE BED READING THE DIRECTIONS ON THE PAIN MEDICATION MACHINE. I WAS SCARED TO DEATH. IT WAS THE MIDDLE OF THE NIGHT, AND I WAS ALONE WITH A NURSE WHO DIDN'T KNOW WHAT SHE WAS DOING.
DR. ROSENBERG CAME IN EARLY AND ASKED HOW I WAS. WHEN I EXPLAINED HOW MY NIGHT WENT, HE BEGAN TO MAKE CALLS.
WHY WOULD WE MOVE A PATIENT FROM INTENSIVE CARE IF WE HAD NO BEDS IN A PROPER SETTING?!
HE HAD ME MOVED IMMEDIATELY TO A SURGICAL FLOOR WITH THE HOSPITAL'S APOLOGIES.

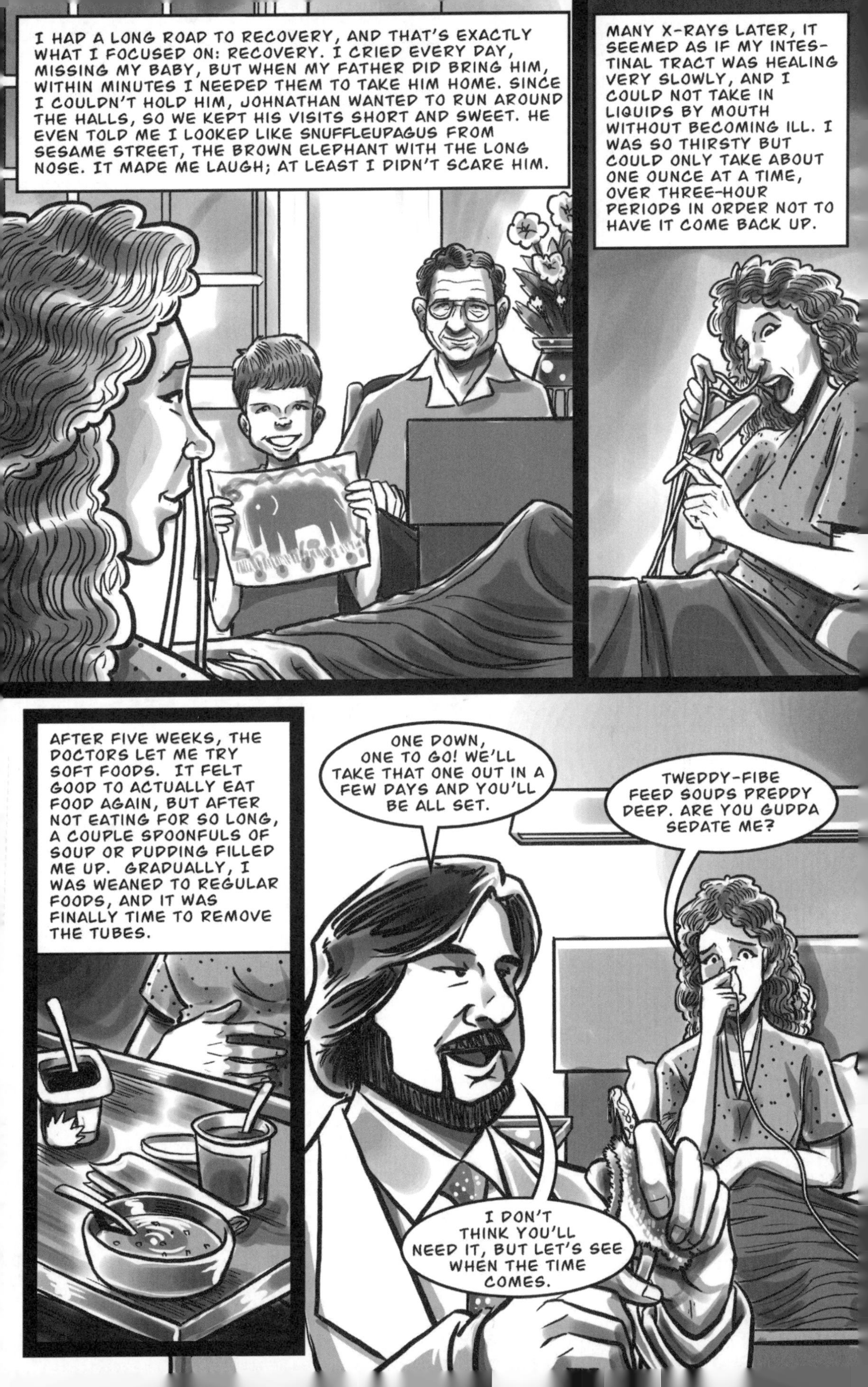
I HAD A LONG ROAD TO RECOVERY, AND THAT'S EXACTLY WHAT I FOCUSED ON: RECOVERY. I CRIED EVERY DAY, MISSING MY BABY, BUT WHEN MY FATHER DID BRING HIM, WITHIN MINUTES I NEEDED THEM TO TAKE HIM HOME. SINCE I COULDN'T HOLD HIM, JOHNATHAN WANTED TO RUN AROUND THE HALLS, SO WE KEPT HIS VISITS SHORT AND SWEET. HE EVEN TOLD ME I LOOKED LIKE SNUFFLEUPAGUS FROM SESAME STREET, THE BROWN ELEPHANT WITH THE LONG NOSE. IT MADE ME LAUGH; AT LEAST I DIDN'T SCARE HIM.
MANY X-RAYS LATER, IT SEEMED AS IF MY INTESTINAL TRACT WAS HEALING VERY SLOWLY, AND I COULD NOT TAKE IN LIQUIDS BY MOUTH WITHOUT BECOMING ILL. I WAS SO THIRSTY BUT COULD ONLY TAKE ABOUT ONE OUNCE AT A TIME, OVER THREE-HOUR PERIODS IN ORDER NOT TO HAVE IT COME BACK UP.
AFTER FIVE WEEKS, THE DOCTORS LET ME TRY SOFT FOODS. IT FELT GOOD TO ACTUALLY EAT FOOD AGAIN, BUT AFTER NOT EATING FOR SO LONG, A COUPLE SPOONFULS OF SOUP OR PUDDING FILLED ME UP. GRADUALLY, I WAS WEANED TO REGULAR FOODS, AND IT WAS FINALLY TIME TO REMOVE THE TUBES.
ONE DOWN, ONE TO GO! WE'LL TAKE THAT ONE OUT IN A FEW DAYS AND YOU'LL BE ALL SET.
TWEDDY-FIBE FEED SOUDS PREDDY DEEP. ARE YOU GUDDA SEDATE ME?
I DON'T THINK YOU'LL NEED IT, BUT LET'S SEE WHEN THE TIME COMES.

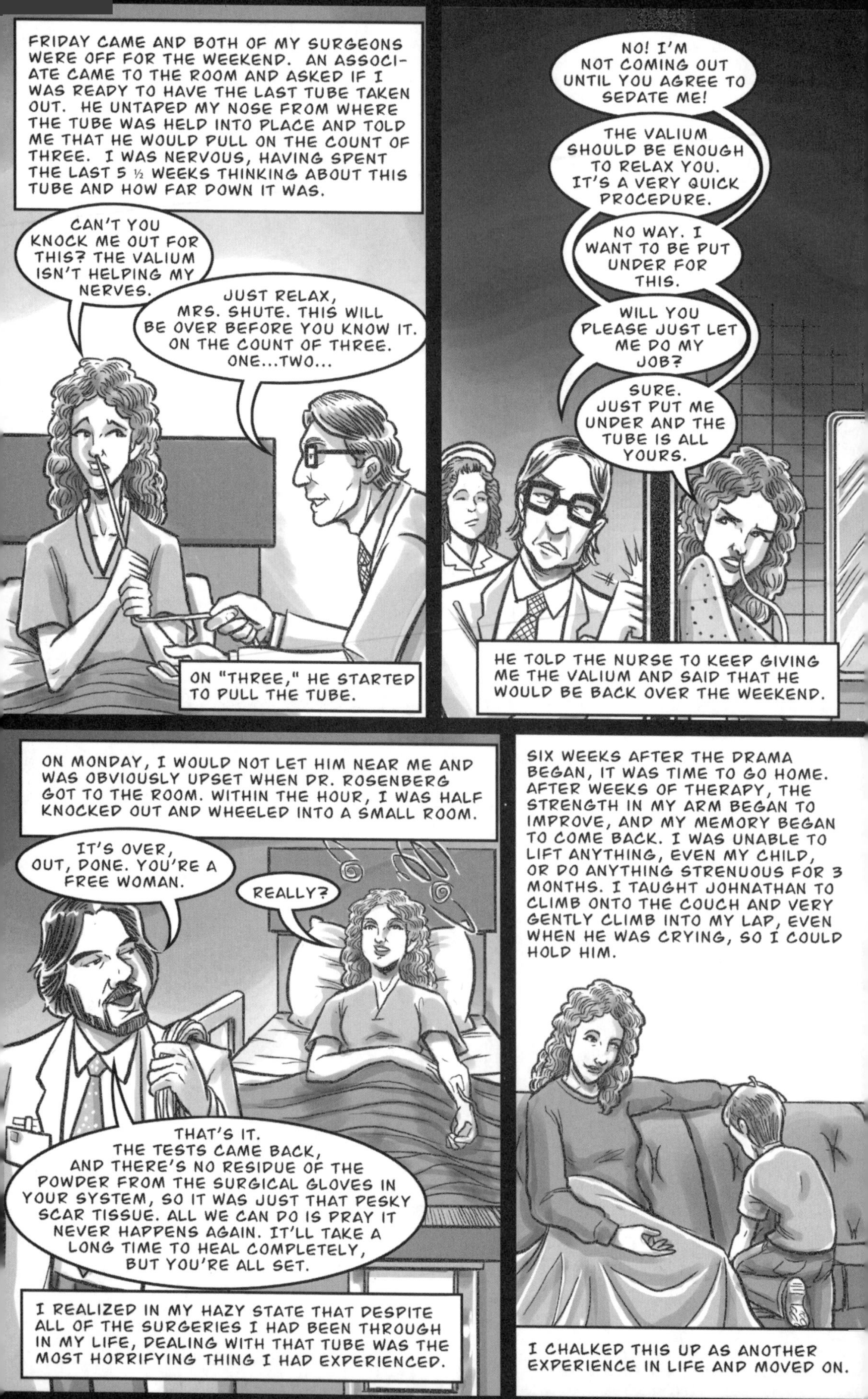
FRIDAY CAME AND BOTH OF MY SURGEONS WERE OFF FOR THE WEEKEND. AN ASSOCIATE CAME TO THE ROOM AND ASKED IF I WAS READY TO HAVE THE LAST TUBE TAKEN OUT. HE UNTAPED MY NOSE FROM WHERE THE TUBE WAS HELD INTO PLACE AND TOLD ME THAT HE WOULD PULL ON THE COUNT OF THREE. I WAS NERVOUS, HAVING SPENT THE LAST 5 ½ WEEKS THINKING ABOUT THIS TUBE AND HOW FAR DOWN IT WAS.
CAN'T YOU KNOCK ME OUT FOR THIS? THE VALIUM ISN'T HELPING MY NERVES.
JUST RELAX, MRS. SHUTE. THIS WILL BE OVER BEFORE YOU KNOW IT. ON THE COUNT OF THREE. ONE...TWO...
ON "THREE," HE STARTED TO PULL THE TUBE.
NO! I'M NOT COMING OUT UNTIL YOU AGREE TO SEDATE ME!
THE VALIUM SHOULD BE ENOUGH TO RELAX YOU. IT'S A VERY QUICK PROCEDURE.
NO WAY. I WANT TO BE PUT UNDER FOR THIS.
WILL YOU PLEASE JUST LET ME DO MY JOB?
SURE. JUST PUT ME UNDER AND THE TUBE IS ALL YOURS.
HE TOLD THE NURSE TO KEEP GIVING ME THE VALIUM AND SAID THAT HE WOULD BE BACK OVER THE WEEKEND.
ON MONDAY, I WOULD NOT LET HIM NEAR ME AND WAS OBVIOUSLY UPSET WHEN DR. ROSENBERG GOT TO THE ROOM. WITHIN THE HOUR, I WAS HALF KNOCKED OUT AND WHEELED INTO A SMALL ROOM.
IT'S OVER, OUT, DONE. YOU'RE A FREE WOMAN.
REALLY?
THAT'S IT. THE TESTS CAME BACK, AND THERE'S NO RESIDUE OF THE POWDER FROM THE SURGICAL GLOVES IN YOUR SYSTEM, SO IT WAS JUST THAT PESKY SCAR TISSUE. ALL WE CAN DO IS PRAY IT NEVER HAPPENS AGAIN. IT'LL TAKE A LONG TIME TO HEAL COMPLETELY, BUT YOU'RE ALL SET.
I REALIZED IN MY HAZY STATE THAT DESPITE ALL OF THE SURGERIES I HAD BEEN THROUGH IN MY LIFE, DEALING WITH THAT TUBE WAS THE MOST HORRIFYING THING I HAD EXPERIENCED.
SIX WEEKS AFTER THE DRAMA BEGAN, IT WAS TIME TO GO HOME. AFTER WEEKS OF THERAPY, THE STRENGTH IN MY ARM BEGAN TO IMPROVE, AND MY MEMORY BEGAN TO COME BACK. I WAS UNABLE TO LIFT ANYTHING, EVEN MY CHILD, OR DO ANYTHING STRENUOUS FOR 3 MONTHS. I TAUGHT JOHNATHAN TO CLIMB ONTO THE COUCH AND VERY GENTLY CLIMB INTO MY LAP, EVEN WHEN HE WAS CRYING, SO I COULD HOLD HIM.
I CHALKED THIS UP AS ANOTHER EXPERIENCE IN LIFE AND MOVED ON.

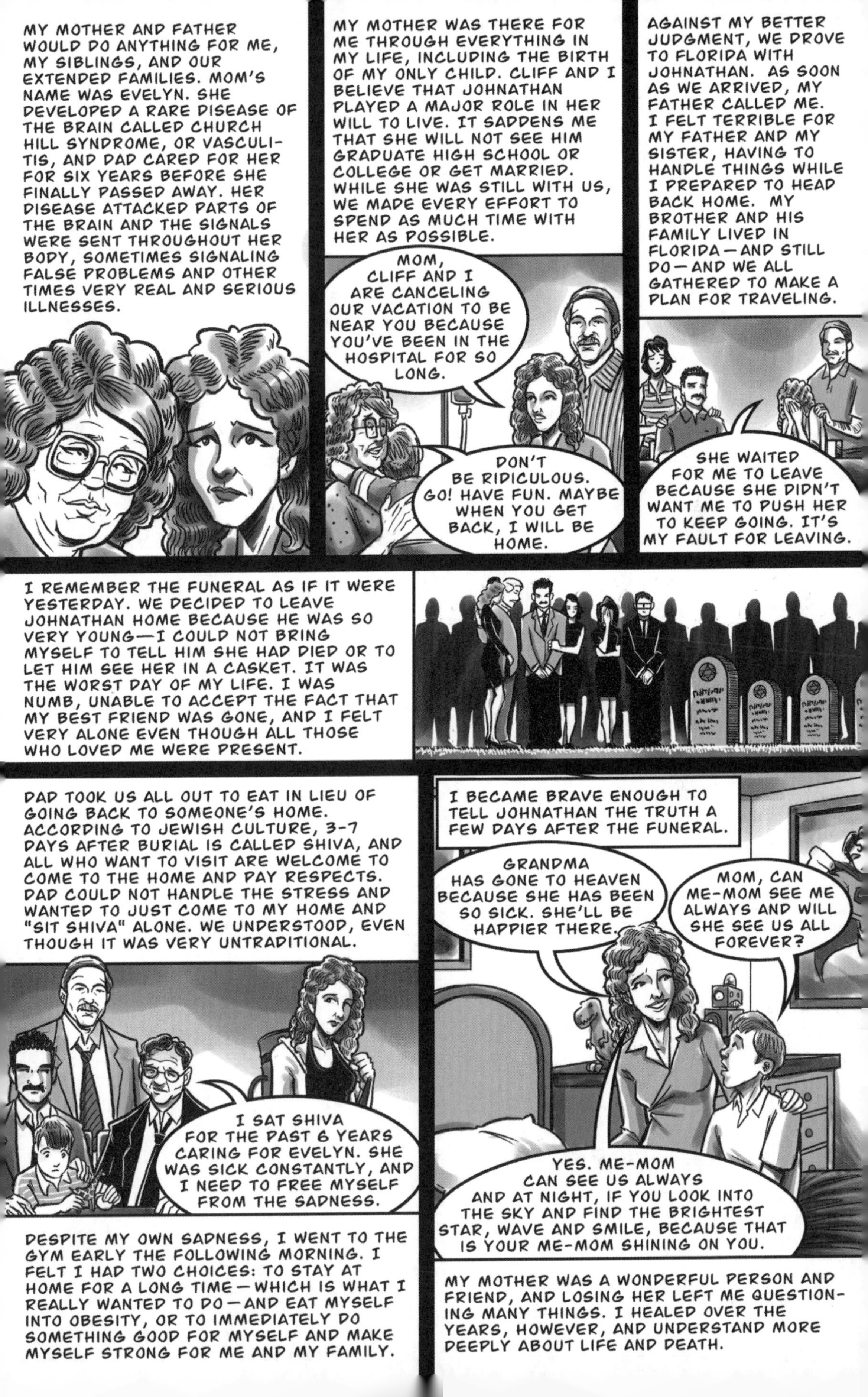
MY MOTHER AND FATHER WOULD DO ANYTHING FOR ME, MY SIBLINGS, AND OUR EXTENDED FAMILIES. MOM'S NAME WAS EVELYN. SHE DEVELOPED A RARE DISEASE OF THE BRAIN CALLED CHURCH HILL SYNDROME, OR VASCULITIS, AND DAD CARED FOR HER FOR SIX YEARS BEFORE SHE FINALLY PASSED AWAY. HER DISEASE ATTACKED PARTS OF THE BRAIN AND THE SIGNALS WERE SENT THROUGHOUT HER BODY, SOMETIMES SIGNALING FALSE PROBLEMS AND OTHER TIMES VERY REAL AND SERIOUS ILLNESSES.
MY MOTHER WAS THERE FOR ME THROUGH EVERYTHING IN MY LIFE, INCLUDING THE BIRTH OF MY ONLY CHILD. CLIFF AND I BELIEVE THAT JOHNATHAN PLAYED A MAJOR ROLE IN HER WILL TO LIVE. IT SADDENS ME THAT SHE WILL NOT SEE HIM GRADUATE HIGH SCHOOL OR COLLEGE OR GET MARRIED. WHILE SHE WAS STILL WITH US, WE MADE EVERY EFFORT TO SPEND AS MUCH TIME WITH HER AS POSSIBLE.
MOM, CLIFF AND I ARE CANCELING OUR VACATION TO BE NEAR YOU BECAUSE YOU'VE BEEN IN THE HOSPITAL FOR SO LONG.
DON'T BE RIDICULOUS. GO! HAVE FUN. MAYBE WHEN YOU GET BACK, I WILL BE HOME.
AGAINST MY BETTER JUDGMENT, WE DROVE TO FLORIDA WITH JOHNATHAN. AS SOON AS WE ARRIVED, MY FATHER CALLED ME. I FELT TERRIBLE FOR MY FATHER AND MY SISTER, HAVING TO HANDLE THINGS WHILE I PREPARED TO HEAD BACK HOME. MY BROTHER AND HIS FAMILY LIVED IN FLORIDA—AND STILL DO—AND WE ALL GATHERED TO MAKE A PLAN FOR TRAVELING.
SHE WAITED FOR ME TO LEAVE BECAUSE SHE DIDN'T WANT ME TO PUSH HER TO KEEP GOING. IT'S MY FAULT FOR LEAVING.
I REMEMBER THE FUNERAL AS IF IT WERE YESTERDAY. WE DECIDED TO LEAVE JOHNATHAN HOME BECAUSE HE WAS SO VERY YOUNG—I COULD NOT BRING MYSELF TO TELL HIM SHE HAD DIED OR TO LET HIM SEE HER IN A CASKET. IT WAS THE WORST DAY OF MY LIFE. I WAS NUMB, UNABLE TO ACCEPT THE FACT THAT MY BEST FRIEND WAS GONE, AND I FELT VERY ALONE EVEN THOUGH ALL THOSE WHO LOVED ME WERE PRESENT.
DAD TOOK US ALL OUT TO EAT IN LIEU OF GOING BACK TO SOMEONE'S HOME. ACCORDING TO JEWISH CULTURE, 3–7 DAYS AFTER BURIAL IS CALLED SHIVA, AND ALL WHO WANT TO VISIT ARE WELCOME TO COME TO THE HOME AND PAY RESPECTS. DAD COULD NOT HANDLE THE STRESS AND WANTED TO JUST COME TO MY HOME AND "SIT SHIVA" ALONE. WE UNDERSTOOD, EVEN THOUGH IT WAS VERY UNTRADITIONAL.
I SAT SHIVA FOR THE PAST 6 YEARS CARING FOR EVELYN. SHE WAS SICK CONSTANTLY, AND I NEED TO FREE MYSELF FROM THE SADNESS.
DESPITE MY OWN SADNESS, I WENT TO THE GYM EARLY THE FOLLOWING MORNING. I FELT I HAD TWO CHOICES: TO STAY AT HOME FOR A LONG TIME—WHICH IS WHAT I REALLY WANTED TO DO—AND EAT MYSELF INTO OBESITY, OR TO IMMEDIATELY DO SOMETHING GOOD FOR MYSELF AND MAKE MYSELF STRONG FOR ME AND MY FAMILY.
I BECAME BRAVE ENOUGH TO TELL JOHNATHAN THE TRUTH A FEW DAYS AFTER THE FUNERAL.
GRANDMA HAS GONE TO HEAVEN BECAUSE SHE HAS BEEN SO SICK. SHE'LL BE HAPPIER THERE.
MOM, CAN ME-MOM SEE ME ALWAYS AND WILL SHE SEE US ALL FOREVER?
YES. ME-MOM CAN SEE US ALWAYS AND AT NIGHT, IF YOU LOOK INTO THE SKY AND FIND THE BRIGHTEST STAR, WAVE AND SMILE, BECAUSE THAT IS YOUR ME-MOM SHINING ON YOU.
MY MOTHER WAS A WONDERFUL PERSON AND FRIEND, AND LOSING HER LEFT ME QUESTIONING MANY THINGS. I HEALED OVER THE YEARS, HOWEVER, AND UNDERSTAND MORE DEEPLY ABOUT LIFE AND DEATH.

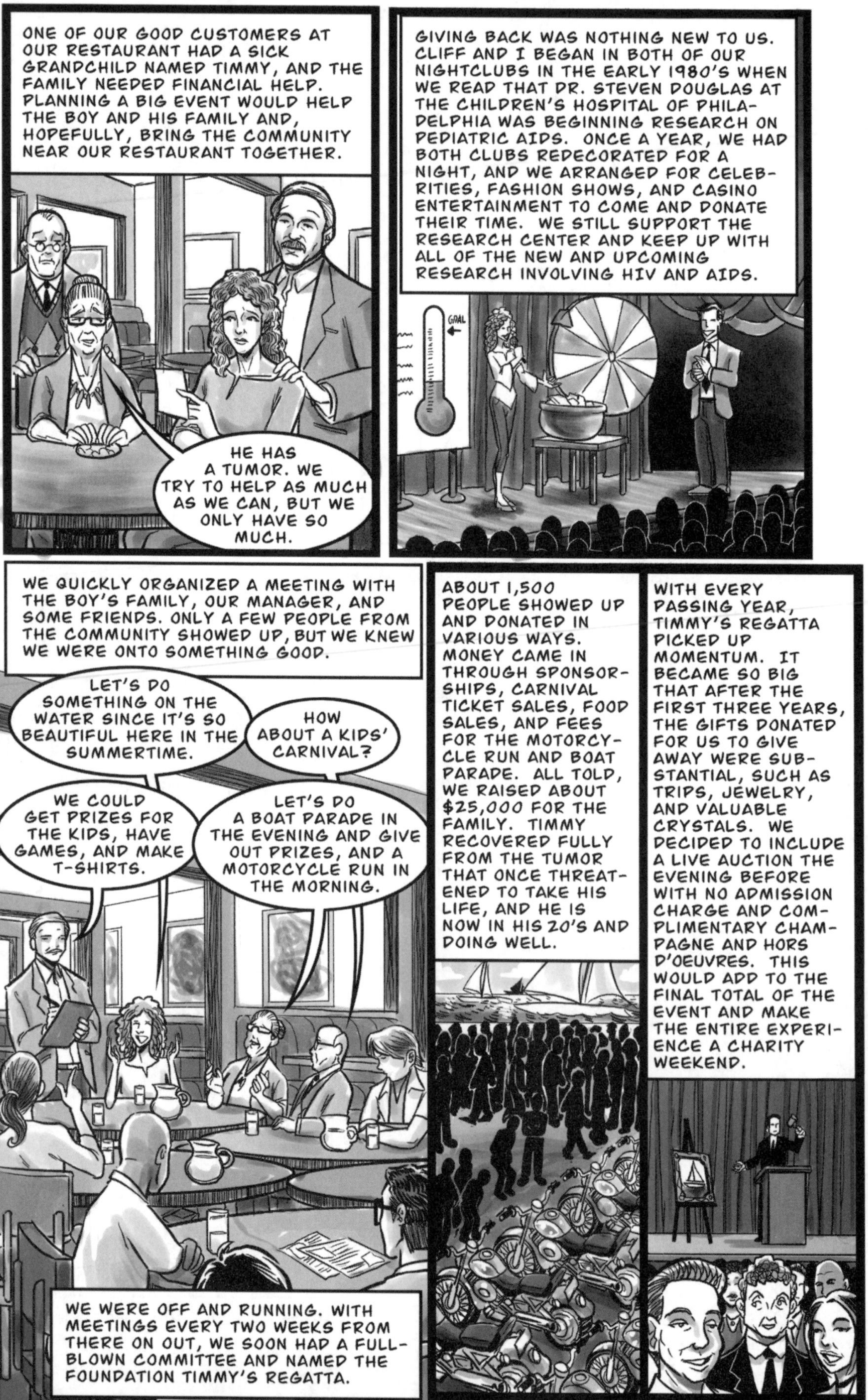
ONE OF OUR GOOD CUSTOMERS AT OUR RESTAURANT HAD A SICK GRANDCHILD NAMED TIMMY, AND THE FAMILY NEEDED FINANCIAL HELP. PLANNING A BIG EVENT WOULD HELP THE BOY AND HIS FAMILY AND, HOPEFULLY, BRING THE COMMUNITY NEAR OUR RESTAURANT TOGETHER.
HE HAS A TUMOR. WE TRY TO HELP AS MUCH AS WE CAN, BUT WE ONLY HAVE SO MUCH.
GIVING BACK WAS NOTHING NEW TO US. CLIFF AND I BEGAN IN BOTH OF OUR NIGHTCLUBS IN THE EARLY 1980'S WHEN WE READ THAT DR. STEVEN DOUGLAS AT THE CHILDREN'S HOSPITAL OF PHILADELPHIA WAS BEGINNING RESEARCH ON PEDIATRIC AIDS. ONCE A YEAR, WE HAD BOTH CLUBS REDECORATED FOR A NIGHT, AND WE ARRANGED FOR CELEBRITIES, FASHION SHOWS, AND CASINO ENTERTAINMENT TO COME AND DONATE THEIR TIME. WE STILL SUPPORT THE RESEARCH CENTER AND KEEP UP WITH ALL OF THE NEW AND UPCOMING RESEARCH INVOLVING HIV AND AIDS.
GOAL
WE QUICKLY ORGANIZED A MEETING WITH THE BOY'S FAMILY, OUR MANAGER, AND SOME FRIENDS. ONLY A FEW PEOPLE FROM THE COMMUNITY SHOWED UP, BUT WE KNEW WE WERE ONTO SOMETHING GOOD.
LET'S DO SOMETHING ON THE WATER SINCE IT'S SO BEAUTIFUL HERE IN THE SUMMERTIME.
HOW ABOUT A KIDS' CARNIVAL?
WE COULD GET PRIZES FOR THE KIDS, HAVE GAMES, AND MAKE T-SHIRTS.
LET'S DO A BOAT PARADE IN THE EVENING AND GIVE OUT PRIZES, AND A MOTORCYCLE RUN IN THE MORNING.
WE WERE OFF AND RUNNING. WITH MEETINGS EVERY TWO WEEKS FROM THERE ON OUT, WE SOON HAD A FULL-BLOWN COMMITTEE AND NAMED THE FOUNDATION TIMMY'S REGATTA.
ABOUT 1,500 PEOPLE SHOWED UP AND DONATED IN VARIOUS WAYS. MONEY CAME IN THROUGH SPONSORSHIPS, CARNIVAL TICKET SALES, FOOD SALES, AND FEES FOR THE MOTORCYCLE RUN AND BOAT PARADE. ALL TOLD, WE RAISED ABOUT $25,000 FOR THE FAMILY. TIMMY RECOVERED FULLY FROM THE TUMOR THAT ONCE THREATENED TO TAKE HIS LIFE, AND HE IS NOW IN HIS 20'S AND DOING WELL.
WITH EVERY PASSING YEAR, TIMMY'S REGATTA PICKED UP MOMENTUM. IT BECAME SO BIG THAT AFTER THE FIRST THREE YEARS, THE GIFTS DONATED FOR US TO GIVE AWAY WERE SUBSTANTIAL, SUCH AS TRIPS, JEWELRY, AND VALUABLE CRYSTALS. WE DECIDED TO INCLUDE A LIVE AUCTION THE EVENING BEFORE WITH NO ADMISSION CHARGE AND COMPLIMENTARY CHAMPAGNE AND HORS D'OEUVRES. THIS WOULD ADD TO THE FINAL TOTAL OF THE EVENT AND MAKE THE ENTIRE EXPERIENCE A CHARITY WEEKEND.

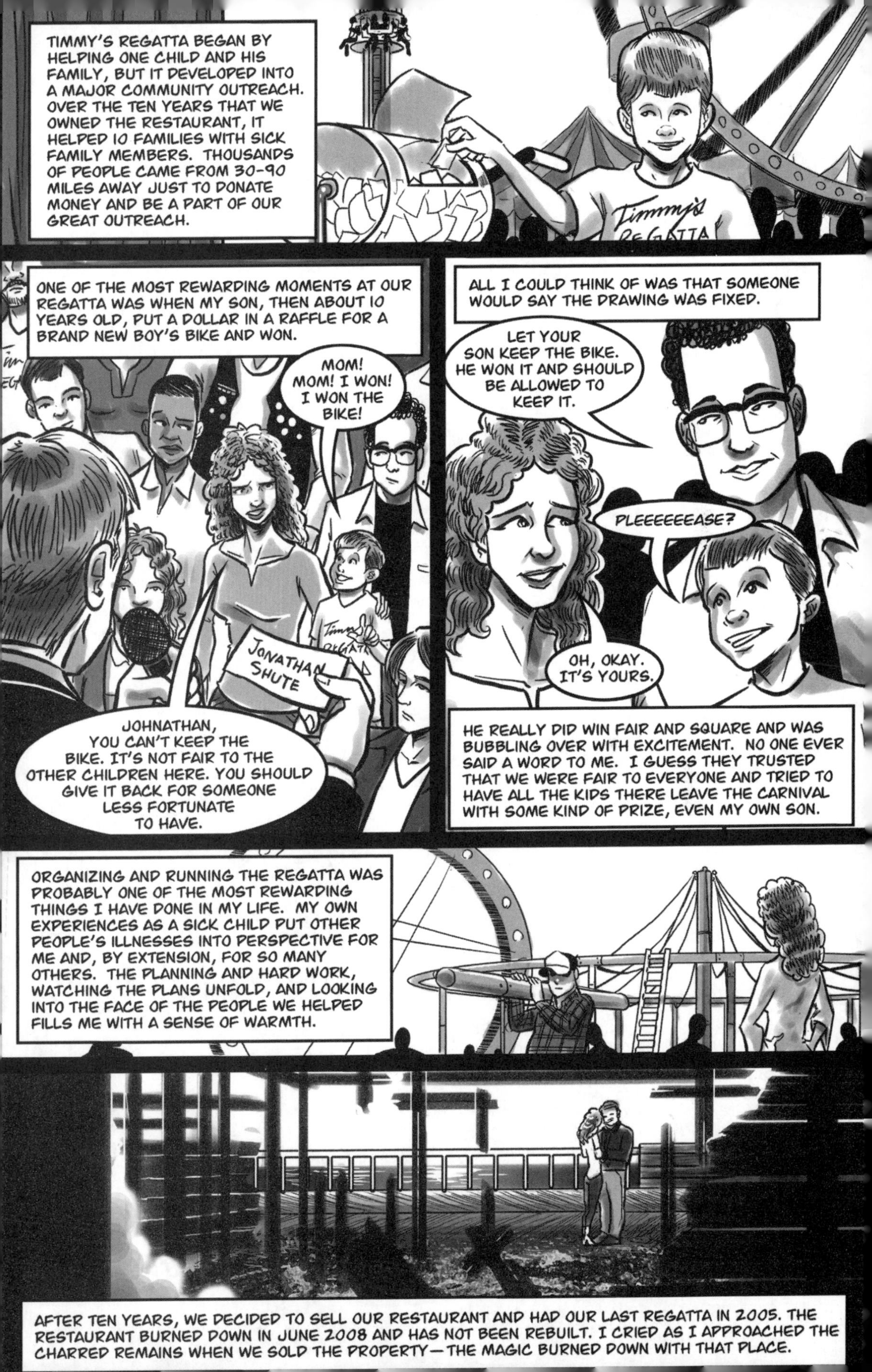
TIMMY'S REGATTA BEGAN BY HELPING ONE CHILD AND HIS FAMILY, BUT IT DEVELOPED INTO A MAJOR COMMUNITY OUTREACH. OVER THE TEN YEARS THAT WE OWNED THE RESTAURANT, IT HELPED 10 FAMILIES WITH SICK FAMILY MEMBERS. THOUSANDS OF PEOPLE CAME FROM 30–90 MILES AWAY JUST TO DONATE MONEY AND BE A PART OF OUR GREAT OUTREACH.
ONE OF THE MOST REWARDING MOMENTS AT OUR REGATTA WAS WHEN MY SON, THEN ABOUT 10 YEARS OLD, PUT A DOLLAR IN A RAFFLE FOR A BRAND NEW BOY'S BIKE AND WON.
MOM! MOM! I WON! I WON THE BIKE!
JONATHAN SHUTE
JOHNATHAN, YOU CAN'T KEEP THE BIKE. IT'S NOT FAIR TO THE OTHER CHILDREN HERE. YOU SHOULD GIVE IT BACK FOR SOMEONE LESS FORTUNATE TO HAVE.
ALL I COULD THINK OF WAS THAT SOMEONE WOULD SAY THE DRAWING WAS FIXED.
LET YOUR SON KEEP THE BIKE. HE WON IT AND SHOULD BE ALLOWED TO KEEP IT.
PLEEEEEEASE?
OH, OKAY. IT'S YOURS.
HE REALLY DID WIN FAIR AND SQUARE AND WAS BUBBLING OVER WITH EXCITEMENT. NO ONE EVER SAID A WORD TO ME. I GUESS THEY TRUSTED THAT WE WERE FAIR TO EVERYONE AND TRIED TO HAVE ALL THE KIDS THERE LEAVE THE CARNIVAL WITH SOME KIND OF PRIZE, EVEN MY OWN SON.
ORGANIZING AND RUNNING THE REGATTA WAS PROBABLY ONE OF THE MOST REWARDING THINGS I HAVE DONE IN MY LIFE. MY OWN EXPERIENCES AS A SICK CHILD PUT OTHER PEOPLE'S ILLNESSES INTO PERSPECTIVE FOR ME AND, BY EXTENSION, FOR SO MANY OTHERS. THE PLANNING AND HARD WORK, WATCHING THE PLANS UNFOLD, AND LOOKING INTO THE FACE OF THE PEOPLE WE HELPED FILLS ME WITH A SENSE OF WARMTH.
AFTER TEN YEARS, WE DECIDED TO SELL OUR RESTAURANT AND HAD OUR LAST REGATTA IN 2005. THE RESTAURANT BURNED DOWN IN JUNE 2008 AND HAS NOT BEEN REBUILT. I CRIED AS I APPROACHED THE CHARRED REMAINS WHEN WE SOLD THE PROPERTY—THE MAGIC BURNED DOWN WITH THAT PLACE.

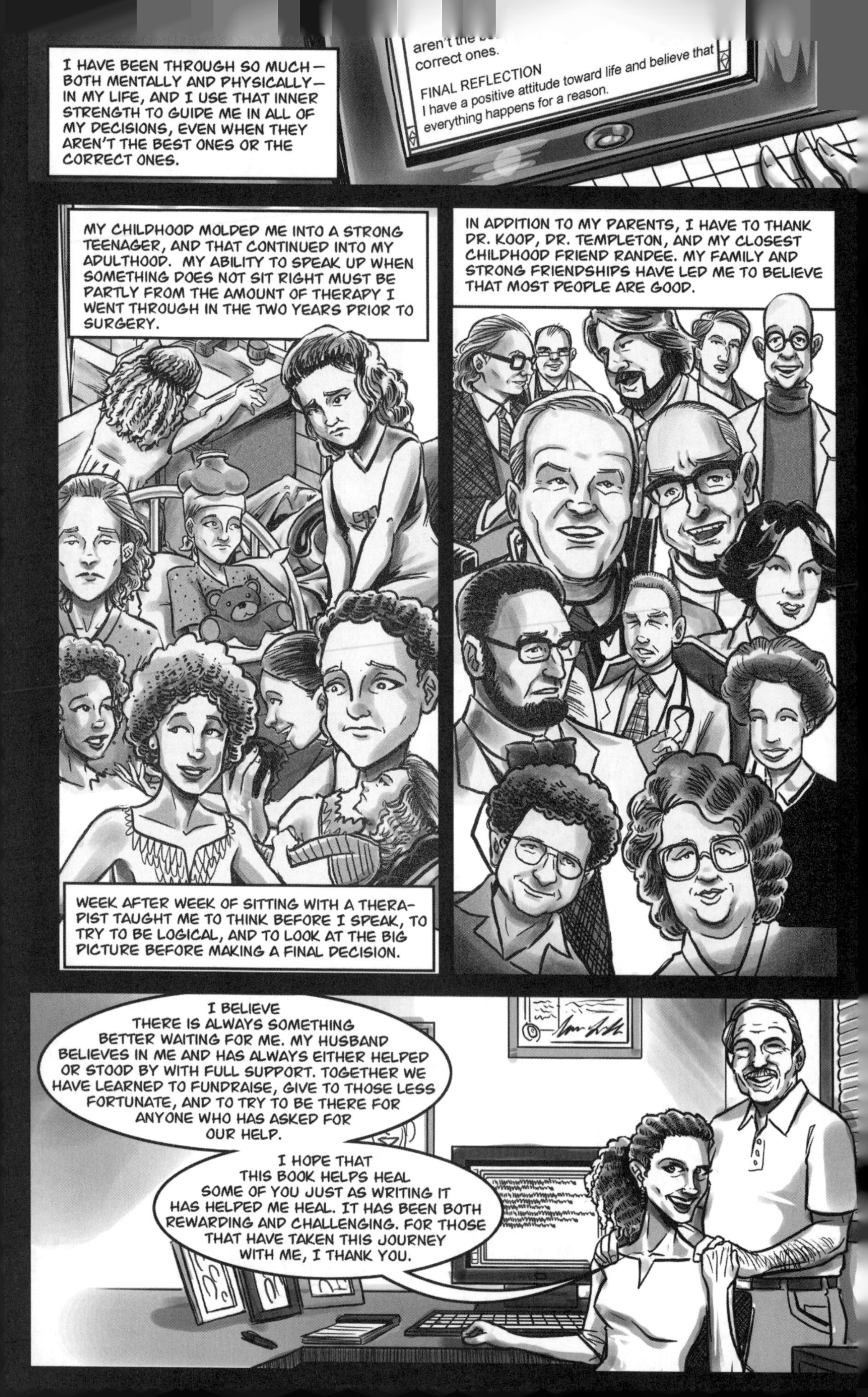
I HAVE BEEN THROUGH SO MUCH—BOTH MENTALLY AND PHYSICALLY—IN MY LIFE, AND I USE THAT INNER STRENGTH TO GUIDE ME IN ALL OF MY DECISIONS, EVEN WHEN THEY AREN'T THE BEST ONES OR THE CORRECT ONES.
correct ones.
FINAL REFLECTION
I have a positive attitude toward life and believe that everything happens for a reason.
MY CHILDHOOD MOLDED ME INTO A STRONG TEENAGER, AND THAT CONTINUED INTO MY ADULTHOOD. MY ABILITY TO SPEAK UP WHEN SOMETHING DOES NOT SIT RIGHT MUST BE PARTLY FROM THE AMOUNT OF THERAPY I WENT THROUGH IN THE TWO YEARS PRIOR TO SURGERY.
WEEK AFTER WEEK OF SITTING WITH A THERAPIST TAUGHT ME TO THINK BEFORE I SPEAK, TO TRY TO BE LOGICAL, AND TO LOOK AT THE BIG PICTURE BEFORE MAKING A FINAL DECISION.
IN ADDITION TO MY PARENTS, I HAVE TO THANK DR. KOOP, DR. TEMPLETON, AND MY CLOSEST CHILDHOOD FRIEND RANDEE. MY FAMILY AND STRONG FRIENDSHIPS HAVE LED ME TO BELIEVE THAT MOST PEOPLE ARE GOOD.
I BELIEVE THERE IS ALWAYS SOMETHING BETTER WAITING FOR ME. MY HUSBAND BELIEVES IN ME AND HAS ALWAYS EITHER HELPED OR STOOD BY WITH FULL SUPPORT. TOGETHER WE HAVE LEARNED TO FUNDRAISE, GIVE TO THOSE LESS FORTUNATE, AND TO TRY TO BE THERE FOR ANYONE WHO HAS ASKED FOR OUR HELP.
I HOPE THAT THIS BOOK HELPS HEAL SOME OF YOU JUST AS WRITING IT HAS HELPED ME HEAL. IT HAS BEEN BOTH REWARDING AND CHALLENGING. FOR THOSE THAT HAVE TAKEN THIS JOURNEY WITH ME, I THANK YOU.

The End

"I DECIDED A LONG TIME AGO THAT I HAD A STORY TO TELL. AS I WROTE IT, I REALIZED I HAD MORE OF A STORY THAN I THOUGHT."

– ALESIA SHUTE, PRESSOFATLANTICCITY.COM

About the Author

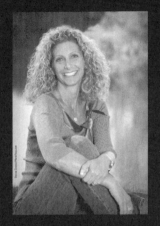

Alesia Shute was born in Philadelphia into a hard working family, and grew up in the Northeast with a dad who worked two jobs and a mom who stayed home with the kids. Alesia dreamed of being a fashion model most of her life, but her height kept her from fully following through. She thought about being a nurse, with her natural compassion for people, but her untimely illness at the age of 7 and subsequent six major surgeries, multiple minor surgeries and long hospital stays made her rethink that career.

In between all of her surgeries, Alesia met her husband, Cliff, whom she has been married to for 28 years. Together they have worked in the nightclub and restaurant business for their entire relationship, balancing marriage and (crazy-all-night, sleep-all-day) work! She helped to raise his daughter, raise their son, and many, many dogs together. They now have two grandchildren from his daughter who give her more love than she could ask for.

Alesia is the proud recipient of the "Good Neighbor Award" for her work on fundraising for a local playground, and she and her husband are active donators to The Children's Hospital of Philadelphia. 'Pediatric Aids Research' is their favorite cause and together they have used their nightclubs as foundations to help raise money to aid the research department and its leading scientist Dr. Steven Douglas in increasing the size of the labs and pursuing many breakthroughs over the past 30 years in Aids Research.

They have used their businesses to hold carnivals and auctions to help families with sick children to pay the bills. Alesia was the president of the Timmy's Regatta Foundation for 10 years and She and Cliff still donate to Ronald McDonald House in Camden New Jersey, as well as to local charities that encourage neighborhood children to participate in sports. All in all, Alesia and Cliff have donated close to one million dollars.

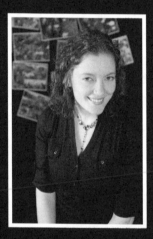

Nadja Baer is the author of several nearly finished fiction novels and the internationally adored webcomic, Impure Blood. Her work has appeared on the kitchen refrigerator, the backs of sales receipts, and at least three crashed hard drives, in addition to several small web and print markets. To her, using big words is both a hobby and a sport. She has been scribbling stories since acquiring her first spiral notebook, but never entertained the thought that someone would pay for her words until her high school English teacher said, "She's going to be a writer some day." Comics and graphic novels have come to hold a special place in her literary nerd's heart, due in large part to cavorting with her illustrator and imminent husband, Nathan Lueth. More insight to their collective psyche can be found by stalking their website at http://www.impurebloodwebcomic.com.

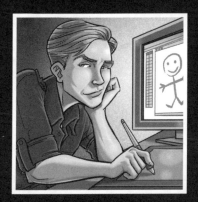

Way back in 1982, Nathan Lueth came into existence with a pencil in his hand. A feat which continues to confound obstetricians to this day. No one knows for sure when he started drawing or where his love of comics came from, but most agree that his professional career began after graduating from the Minneapolis College of Art and Design, as a caricaturist in the Mall of America. Soon he was freelance illustrating for the likes of Target, General Mills, and Picture Window Books. He is proud to be a part of Writers of the Round Table as he believes that comics should be for everyone, not just nerds (it should be noted that he may be trying to turn the general population into nerds). He currently resides in St. Paul, MN, with a cat, a turtle, and his imminent wife, Nadja, upon whom he performs his nerd conversion experiments.

CHILD ALESIA

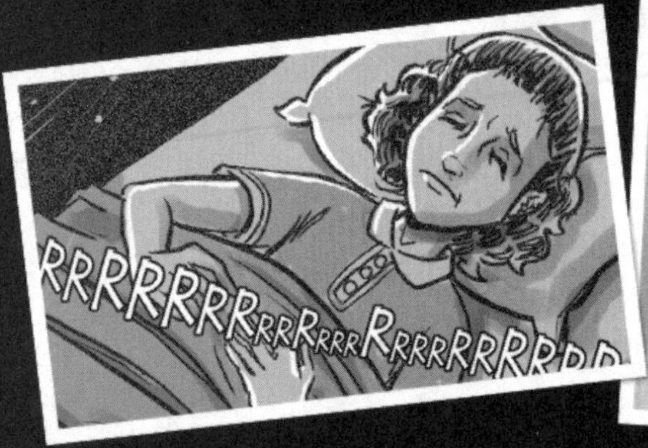

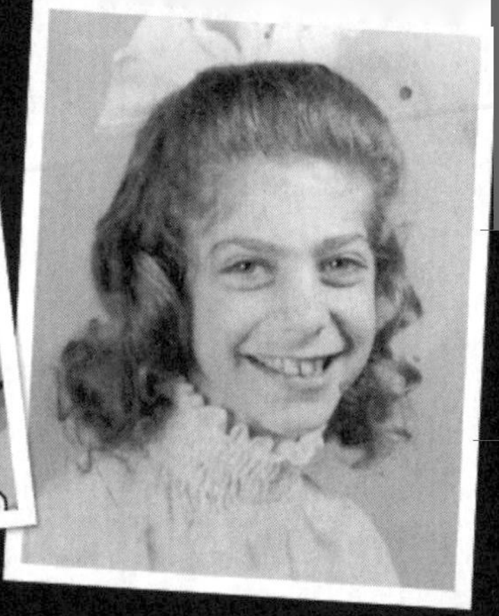

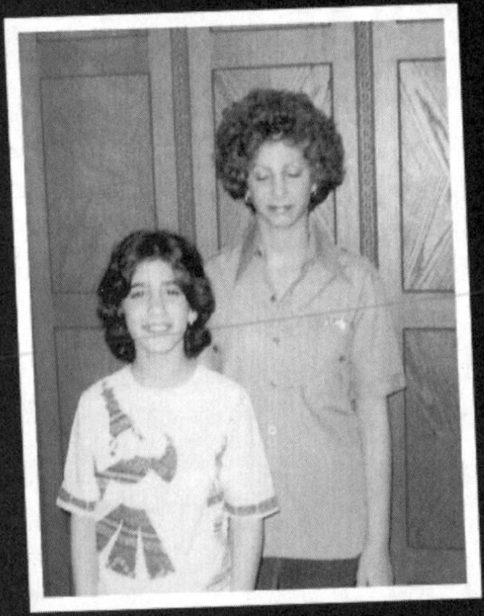

TEENAGE ALES

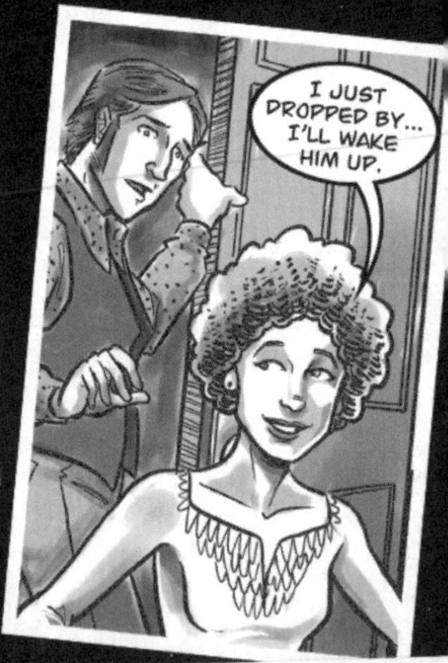
I JUST DROPPED BY... I'LL WAKE HIM UP.

ADULT ALESIA

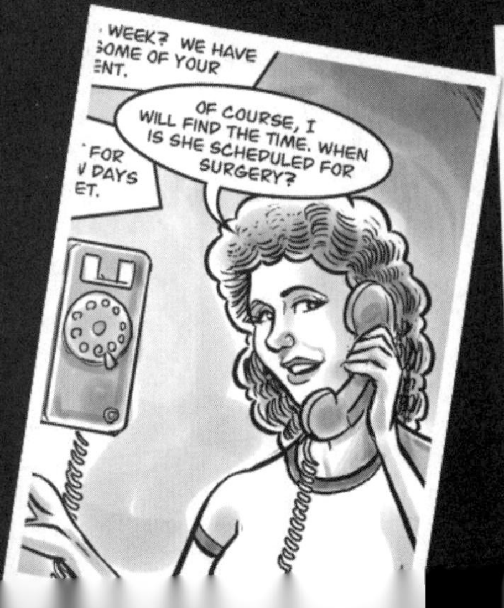
OF COURSE, I WILL FIND THE TIME. WHEN IS SHE SCHEDULED FOR SURGERY?

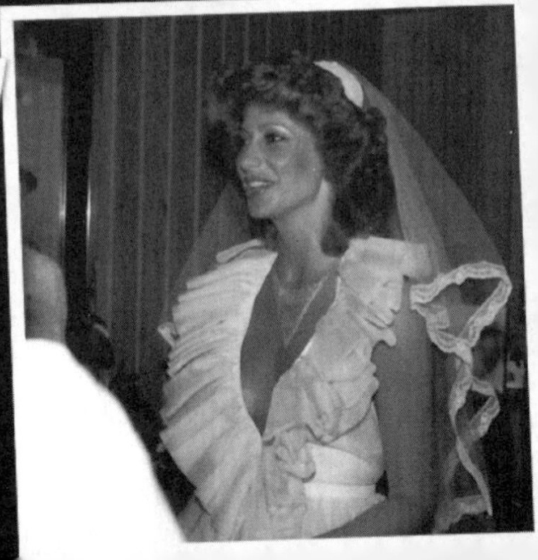

ALESIA'S PARENTS

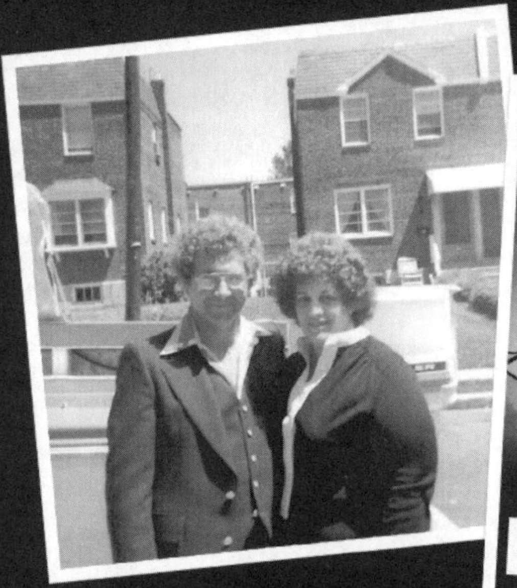

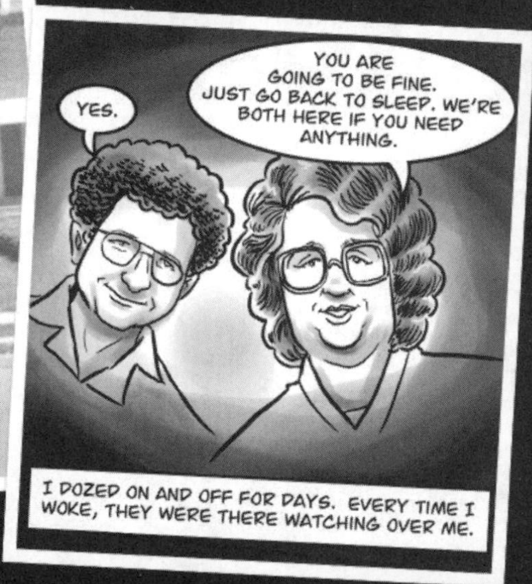
YES.
YOU ARE GOING TO BE FINE. JUST GO BACK TO SLEEP. WE'RE BOTH HERE IF YOU NEED ANYTHING.
I DOZED ON AND OFF FOR DAYS. EVERY TIME I WOKE, THEY WERE THERE WATCHING OVER ME.

ALESIA'S MOM

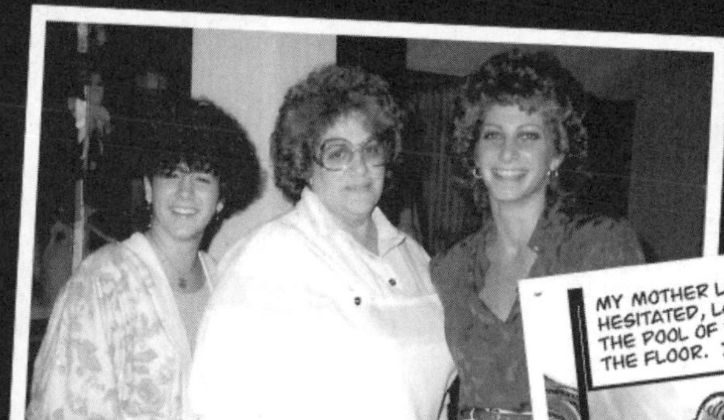

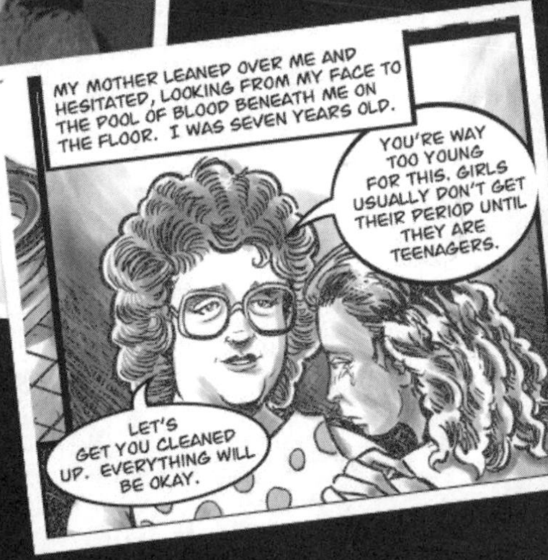
MY MOTHER LEANED OVER ME AND HESITATED, LOOKING FROM MY FACE TO THE POOL OF BLOOD BENEATH ME ON THE FLOOR. I WAS SEVEN YEARS OLD.
YOU'RE WAY TOO YOUNG FOR THIS. GIRLS USUALLY DON'T GET THEIR PERIOD UNTIL THEY ARE TEENAGERS.
LET'S GET YOU CLEANED UP. EVERYTHING WILL BE OKAY.

ALESIA'S DAD

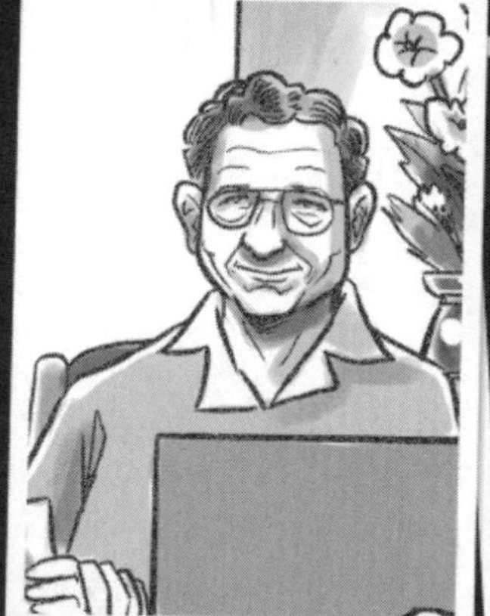

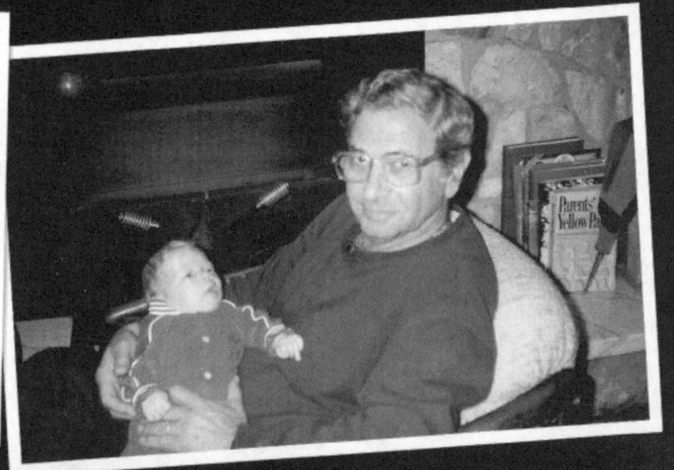

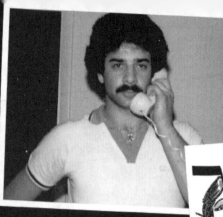

ALESIA'S
BROTHER

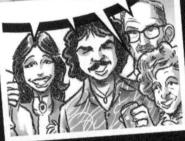

CLIFF'S
PARENTS

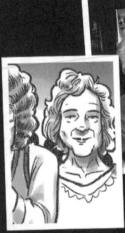

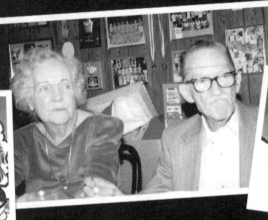

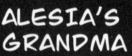

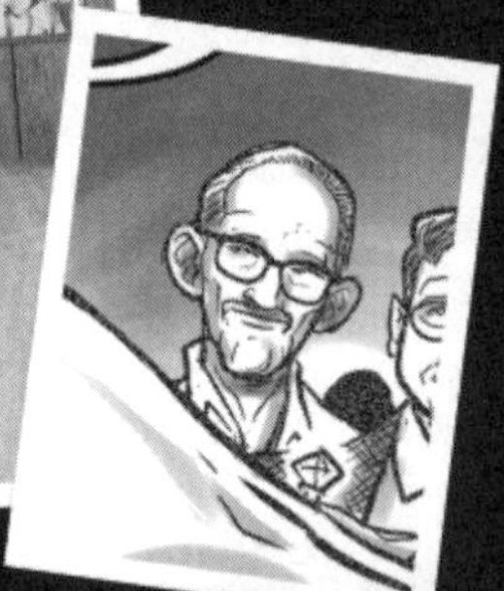

ALESIA'S
GRANDMA

IT'S GOOD
LUCK. WELCOME TO
WOMANHOOD!

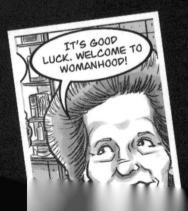

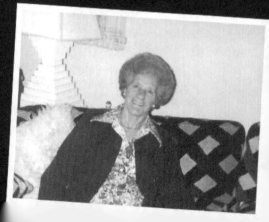

ALESIA'S SISTER

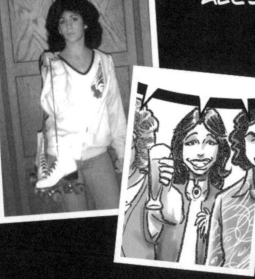

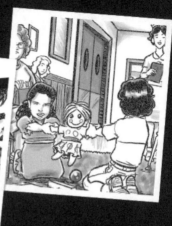

ALESIA'S GIRLFRIEND TERRY

A BIT LATER, CLIFF CAME BACK AND HANDED A BIG BAG TO MY GIRLFRIEND, TERRY.
OH GREAT! SHRIMP! EVERYONE WILL GO CRAZY! WAIT A SECOND... WHAT DO WE DO WITH THESE? THEY STILL HAVE THEIR HEADS ON.
NO BIG DEAL, JUST PEEL THEM OFF.

CAN
PIT. CAN'T
GRAB IT
PULL IT
INTO YOUR STOMA, BUT
HAVE TO
MY
PHIA.
THE
THEY

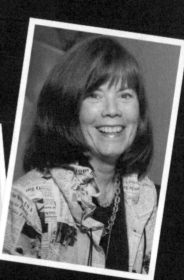

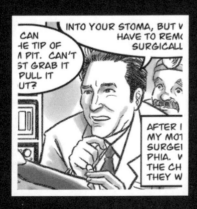

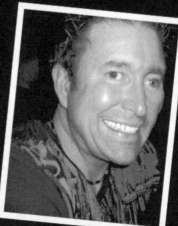

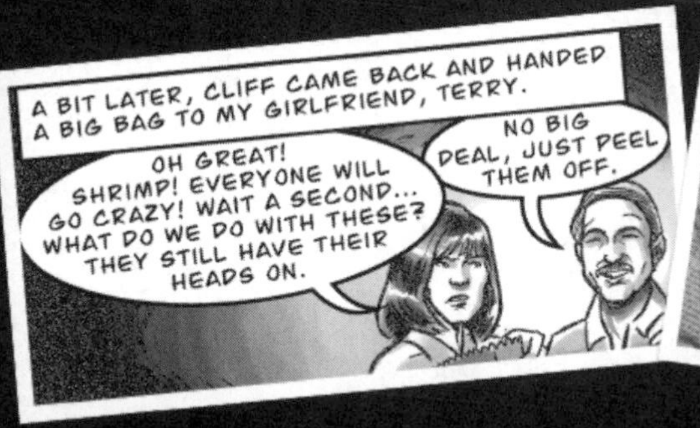

CONTEST WINNER
CHRIS FLICKENGER

CLIFF

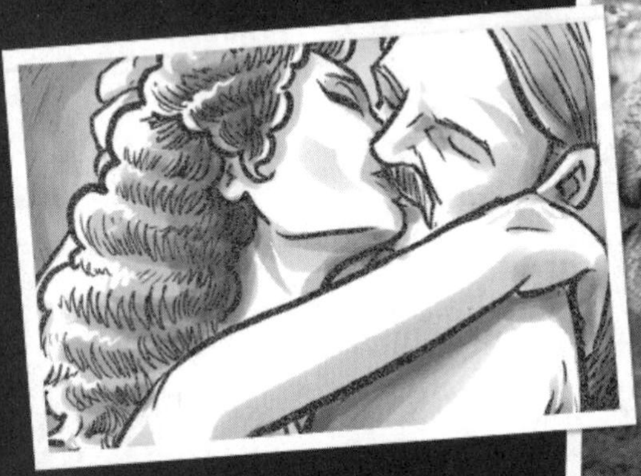

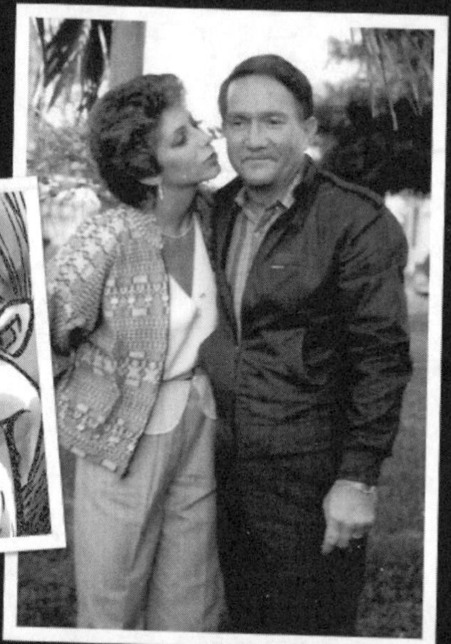

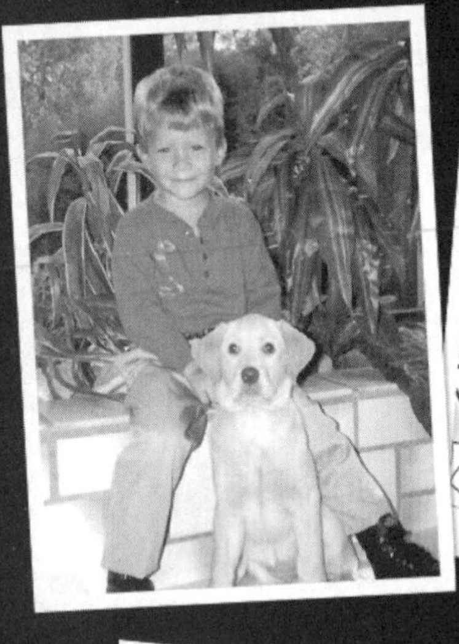

JOHNATHAN

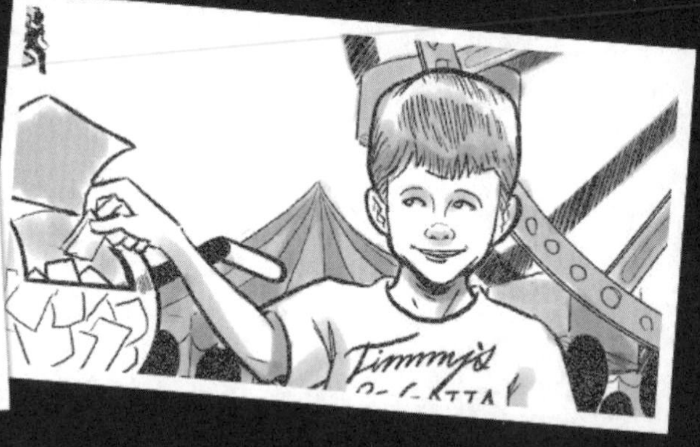
Timmy's

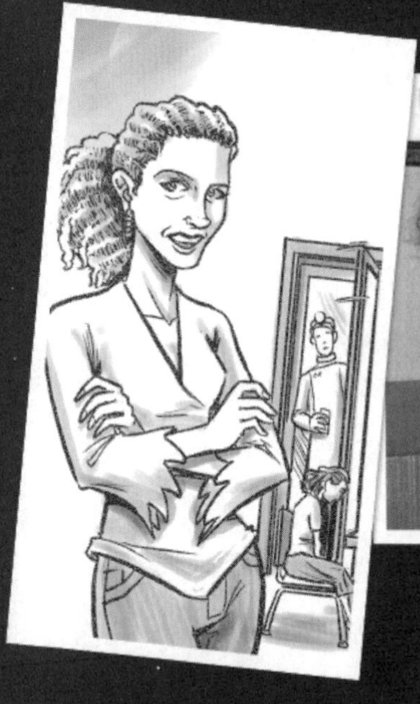

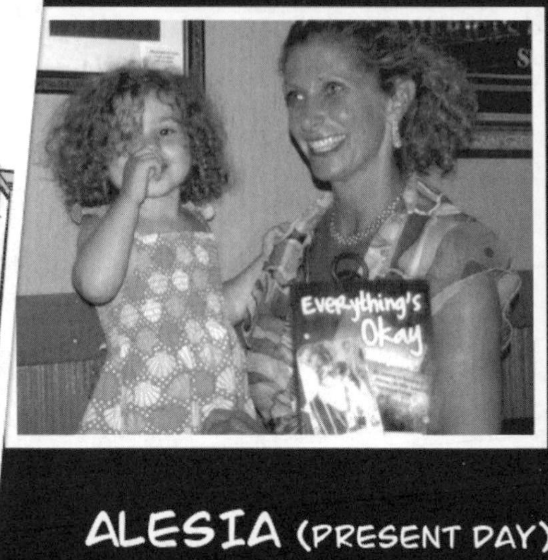
Everything's
Okay

ALESIA (PRESENT DAY)

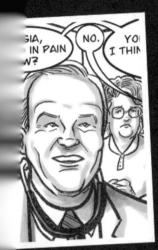

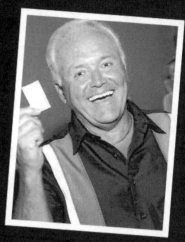

BRENT LILLISTON

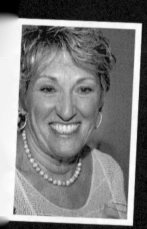

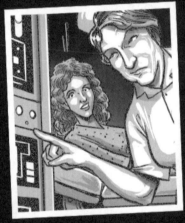

NANCY BARTLE

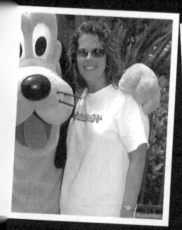

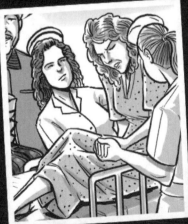

ALESTA'S COUSIN LAURA

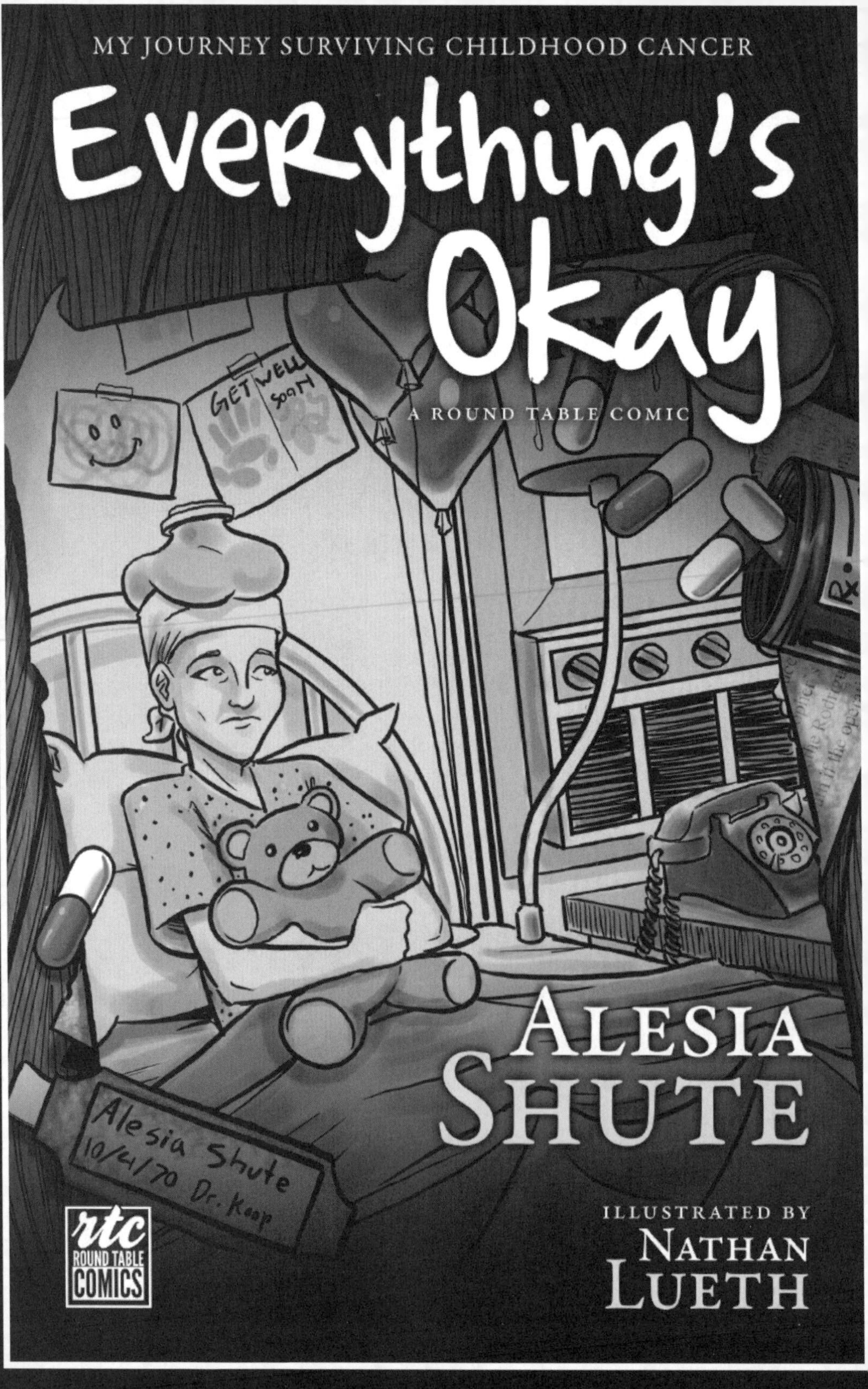

MY JOURNEY SURVIVING CHILDHOOD CANCER
Everything's Okay
A ROUND TABLE COMIC
GET WELL soon
Rx
Alesia Shute 10/4/70 Dr. Koop
ALESIA SHUTE
rtc ROUND TABLE COMICS
ILLUSTRATED BY
NATHAN LUETH

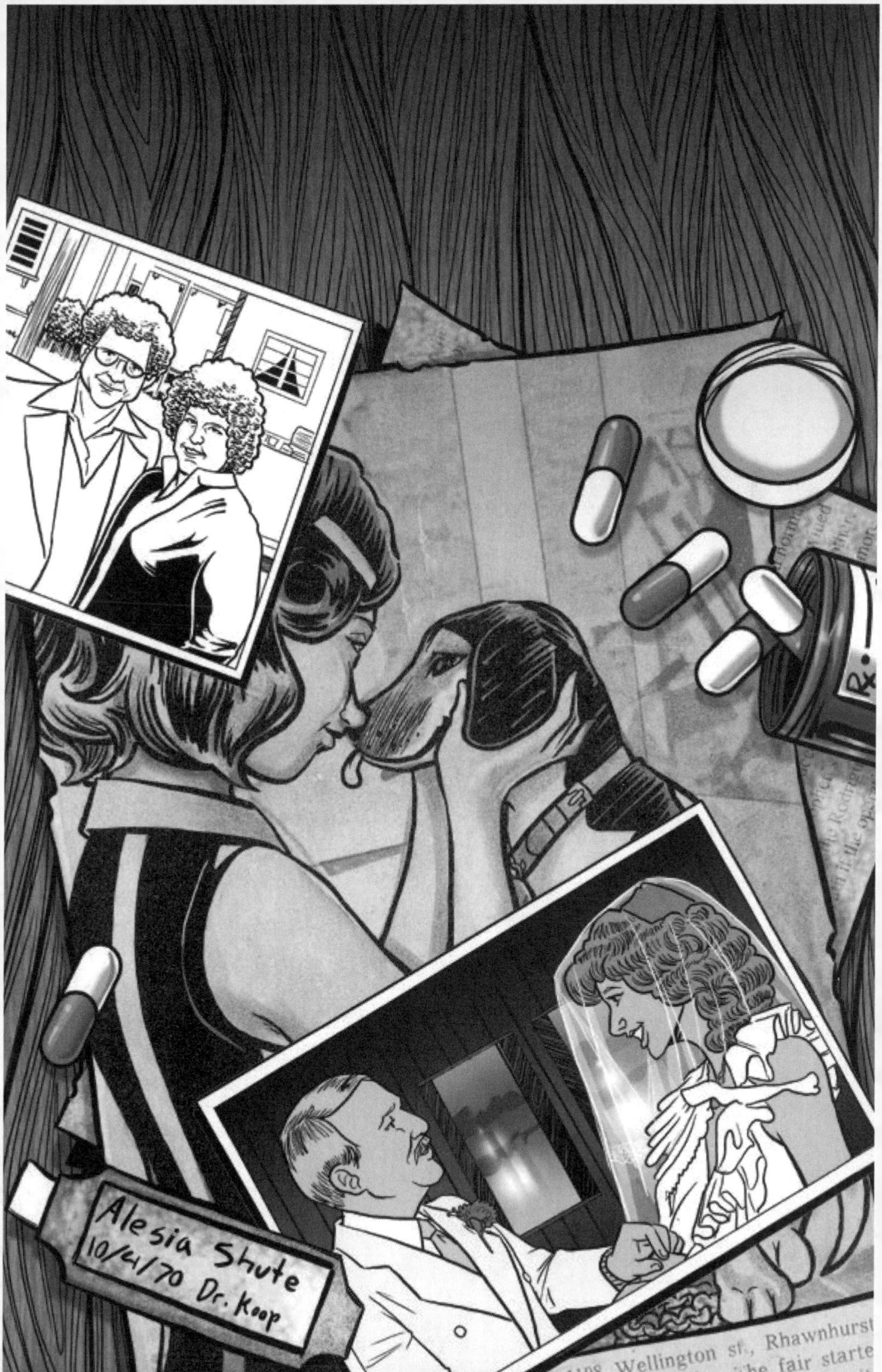
Alesia Shute
10/4/70 Dr. Koop
of 1108 Wellington st., Rhawnhurst

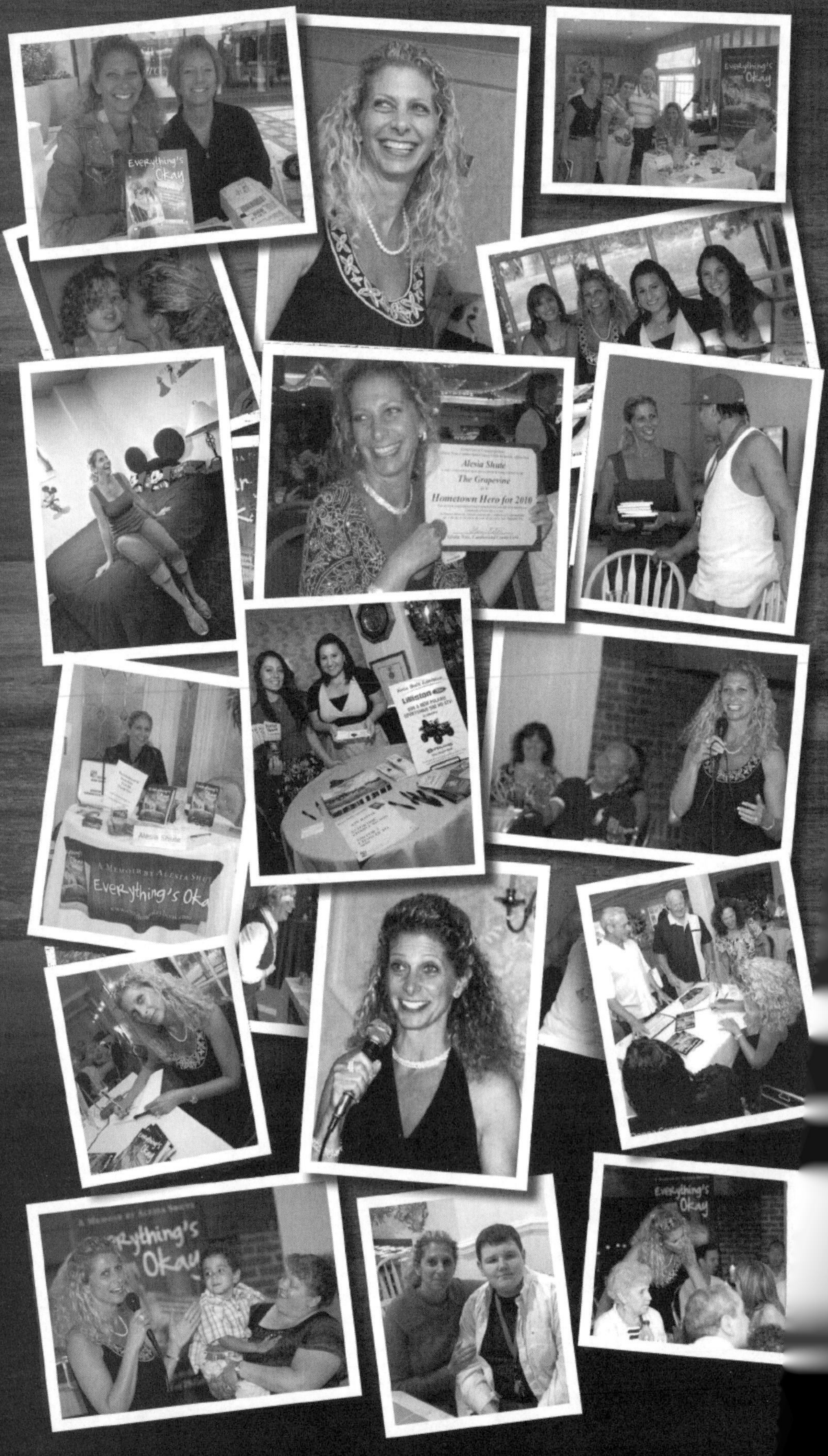
Everything's Okay
Everything's Okay
Alesia Shute
The Grapevine
Hometown Hero for 2010
Alesia Shute
A Memoir by Alesia Shute
Everything's Okay
Everything's Okay
Everything's Okay

Alesia Shute Foundation

The mission of the Alesia Shute Foundation is to improve the lives of families facing childhood disease, both by making hospital stays more comfortable and by funding the research that will treat or eliminate childhood illnesses. Alesia Shute's recount of her own battle and triumph over childhood cancer in her book, Everything's Okay, was written to inform and encourage families struggling to survive through childhood illness. Donations to the Alesia Shute Foundation go towards the delivery of Alesia's books to families in need. Profits from the book sales are donated directly to The Children's Hospital of Philadelphia (CHOP). The Alesia Shute Foundation is recognized in NJ as a not-for-profit company.

A REMARKABLE JOURNEY THROUGH THE EYES OF A CHILD WHO FACED ADVERSITY AND SCOFFED AT IT. SHE [THE AUTHOR] WAS WISE BEYOND HER YEARS AND WITH THE SUPPORT OF AN EXCEPTIONAL FAMILY, SHE WAS ABLE TO OVERCOME THE CHALLENGES OF LIVING WITH A CHRONIC AND DISABLING CONDITION. A BOOK FOR PATIENTS AND FAMILY MEMBERS WHO NEED TO SEE THAT THERE IS ALWAYS LIGHT AT THE END OF THE TUNNEL."
- JENIFER, MOTHER OF A CHILD BATTLING CROHN'S DISEASE

AS I READ THE BOOK I FELT AS IF I WAS THERE WITH ALESIA AND KEPT THINKING HOW BRAVE SHE WAS. THROUGHOUT MY TEACHING CAREER I HAVE HAD STUDENTS THAT HAVE BEEN DIAGNOSED WITH SERIOUS ILLNESSES AND WISH I HAD A BOOK LIKE THIS ONE TO RECOMMEND TO THEIR PARENTS. IT GIVES HOPE, WHICH IS SOMETHING FAMILIES DESPERATELY NEED AT SUCH A TIME. EVERYTHING'S OKAY MAKES THE READER REALIZE THAT THERE ARE THINGS WE CAN AND CAN'T CONTROL AND IT REMINDS US TO APPRECIATE EVERYTHING THAT IS GOOD IN OUR LIVES." - ESTHER GOLDBLATT, TEACHER

"WHAT TYPE OF WORK IS THE MOST REWARDING AND SATISFYING? GIVING BACK. HELPING OTHERS." – ALESIA SHUTE, AKGMAG.COM

CONTACT:

ALESIA@EVERYTHINGSOKAYBOOK.COM
WWW.EVERYTHINGSOKAYBOOK.COM
501(C)3: 27-0601335

Media Inquiries
Amy Toosley
Allison & Partners
roundtable@allisonspr.com

Speaking Engagements
Erin Cohen
815.301.9546
erin@roundtablecompanies.com

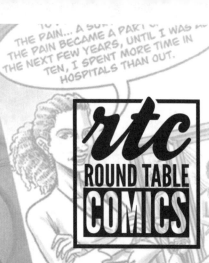

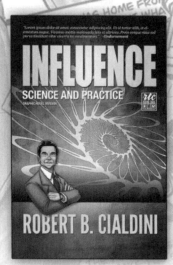

COMING SOON FROM ROUND TABLE COMICS

FOR THOSE WHO LEAD IN BUSINESS
AND THOSE WHO LEAD IN LIFE
EDGE!
A LEADERSHIP STORY
Bea Fields
Corey Michael Blake
WITH EVA SILVA TRAVERS
Illustrated by Nathan Lueth
WITH A FOREWORD
BY MICHAEL E. GERBER,
AUTHOR OF THE E-MYTH BOOKS

INFLUENCE
SCIENCE AND PRACTICE
ROBERT B. CIALDINI

the ALTUCHER
CONFIDENTIAL
IDEAS FOR A WORLD OUT OF BALANCE
JAMES
ALTUCHER
ILLUSTRATED BY
TBD

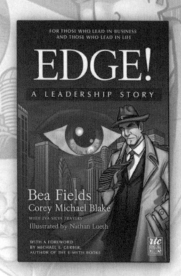

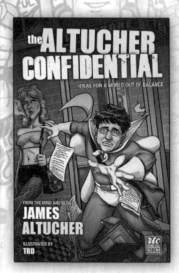

For more information visit:
www.roundtablecompanies.com

Follow us:
@RndTableCompanies

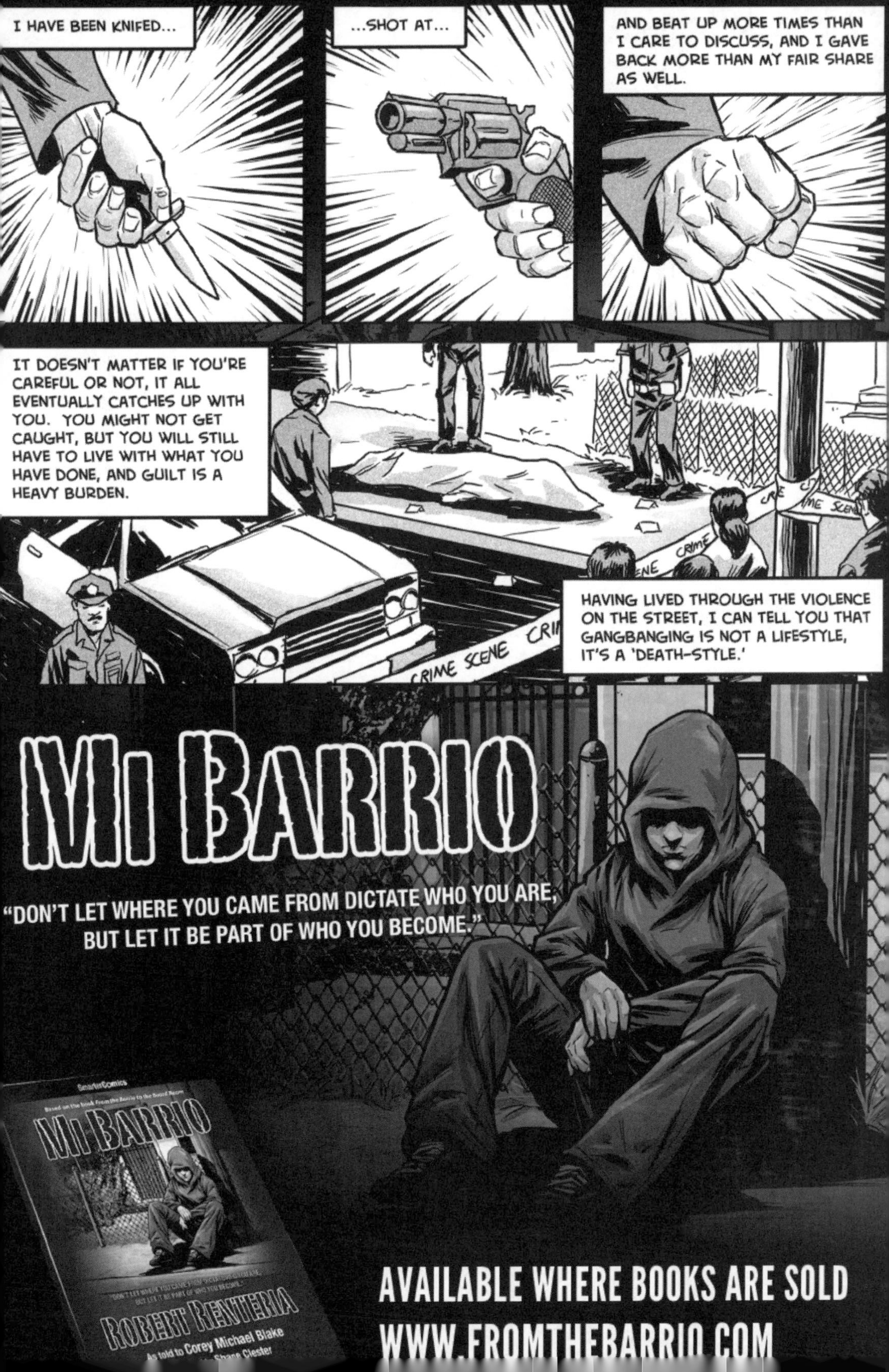
I HAVE BEEN KNIFED...
...SHOT AT...
AND BEAT UP MORE TIMES THAN I CARE TO DISCUSS, AND I GAVE BACK MORE THAN MY FAIR SHARE AS WELL.
IT DOESN'T MATTER IF YOU'RE CAREFUL OR NOT, IT ALL EVENTUALLY CATCHES UP WITH YOU. YOU MIGHT NOT GET CAUGHT, BUT YOU WILL STILL HAVE TO LIVE WITH WHAT YOU HAVE DONE, AND GUILT IS A HEAVY BURDEN.
CRIME SCENE
HAVING LIVED THROUGH THE VIOLENCE ON THE STREET, I CAN TELL YOU THAT GANGBANGING IS NOT A LIFESTYLE, IT'S A 'DEATH-STYLE.'
MI BARRIO
"DON'T LET WHERE YOU CAME FROM DICTATE WHO YOU ARE, BUT LET IT BE PART OF WHO YOU BECOME."
MI BARRIO
ROBERT RENTERIA
As told to Corey Michael Blake
AVAILABLE WHERE BOOKS ARE SOLD
WWW.FROMTHEBARRIO.COM

HOW SUCCESSFUL PEOPLE BECOME
EVEN MORE SUCCESSFUL

WHAT GOT YOU HERE WON'T GET YOU THERE

DISCOVER THE 20 WORKPLACE HABITS THAT YOU NEED TO BREAK

MARSHALL GOLDSMITH

WITH MARK REITER

ILLUSTRATED BY
SHANE CLESTER

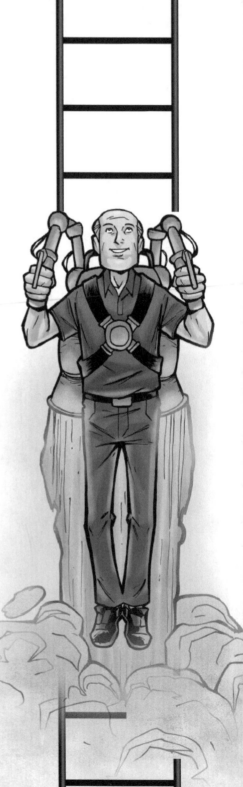